"This group of experts is to be commended for writing such an accessible and t
challenging transitional period in women's lives. Melding state-of-the-art resea
clinical wisdom, this workbook teaches readers effective cognitive behavioral s
moods and sustaining their engagement with meaningful life choices during menopause."

—Zindel V. Segal, author of *The Mindful Way through Depression*

"This book details crucial information for every woman nearing or experiencing menopause, providing the reader with basic knowledge of processes associated with this transitional period of life and guiding her to discovery of effective personalized symptom management and coping strategies. The content is excellent. The language is accessible. The strategies are evidence based and engaging. Positive outcomes await the reader."

—Gordon J. G. Asmundson, PhD, RD, CACBT, professor of psychology and editor-in-chief of *Cognitive Behaviour Therapy* (cognbehavther.com)

The Cognitive Behavioral Workbook *for* Menopause

A STEP-BY-STEP PROGRAM *for* OVERCOMING HOT FLASHES, MOOD SWINGS, INSOMNIA, ANXIETY, DEPRESSION, *and* OTHER SYMPTOMS

SHERYL M. GREEN, PhD
RANDI E. M^cCABE, PhD
CLAUDIO N. SOARES, MD, PhD

New Harbinger Publications, Inc.

Publisher's Note

This publication is designed to provide accurate and authoritative information in regard to the subject matter covered. It is sold with the understanding that the publisher is not engaged in rendering psychological, financial, legal, or other professional services. If expert assistance or counseling is needed, the services of a competent professional should be sought.

Distributed in Canada by Raincoast Books

Copyright © 2012 by Sheryl M. Green, Randi E. McCabe, and Claudio N. Soares
New Harbinger Publications, Inc.
5674 Shattuck Avenue
Oakland, CA 94609
www.newharbinger.com

All Rights Reserved

Acquired by Melissa Kirk; Cover design by Amy Shoup; Edited by Brady Kahn; Text design by Tracy Carlson

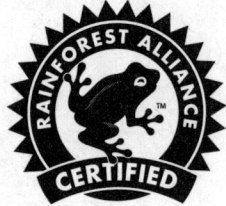

Library of Congress Cataloging-in-Publication Data

Green, Sheryl M.
  The cognitive behavioral workbook for menopause : a step-by-step program for overcoming hot flashes, mood swings, insomnia, anxiety, depression and other symptoms / Sheryl M. Green, Randi E. McCabe, and Claudio Soares.
    p. cm.
  Includes bibliographical references.
  ISBN 978-1-60882-110-5 (pbk. : alk. paper) -- ISBN 978-1-60882-111-2 (pdf e-book) -- ISBN 978-1-60882-112-9 (epub) 1. Menopause--Treatment--Popular works. 2. Cognitive therapy--Popular works. 3. Women--Health and hygiene. 4. Self-care, Health--Popular works. I. McCabe, Randi E. II. Soares, Claudio N. III. Title.
  RG186.G727 2012
  618.1'7506--dc23

                            2012021955

Printed in the United States of America

14 13 12   10 9 8 7 6 5 4 3 2 1   First printing

For my ever precious daughters:
Claire Addison Green Kopeck and Ana Cole Green Kopeck

–S. M. G.

For my boys:
Will, Liam, Brendan, and Casey

–R. E. M.

For my wife Christy and for all my patients for sharing their stories and guiding me through their experiences

–C. N. S.

Contents

Foreword vii

Acknowledgments ix

Introduction 1

PART 1
Menopause, Its Symptoms, and Your Treatment Options

1   Learning about Menopause 7

2   Recognizing Your Symptoms 17

3   Choosing among the Treatment Options 27

4   Taking a Cognitive Behavioral Approach 35

PART 2
Cognitive Behavioral Treatment for Menopausal Symptoms

5   Managing Hot Flashes and Night Sweats 53

6   Coping with Anxiety 73

7   Dealing with Depression and Other Feelings 97

8   Getting a Good Night's Sleep 125

9   Addressing Urogenital Problems and Sexual Concerns 145

10   Consolidating Your Gains and Moving Forward 165

    Suggested Reading 175

    References 177

Foreword

Menopause is a time of transition. For most women, it begins five to ten years after midlife and lasts an average of four years. It is a time of hormonal change, and it represents the natural transition from a reproductive to a nonreproductive phase of life. Yet, this change does not occur without announcing itself with a range of signs and symptoms. In the first phase, the natural waxing and waning of hormones across the monthly cycle becomes more erratic, and with these changes comes a host of symptoms that prominently include hot flashes, night sweats, sleeping difficulties, mood swings, and challenges to sexual functioning and enjoyment. As the body transitions further toward full menopause, the menstrual cycle may be missed for two or more months, and symptoms may intensify from the early soft notes of change to a fuller orchestra of symptoms proclaiming your transition to postmenopausal life. And while this change of life is as natural as the sun passing across the sky, the timing, intensity, and degree of impairment of the accompanying symptoms may not strike any two women alike. To meet the challenge of the menopausal transition, an individualized approach to coping with symptoms is needed.

This individualized approach is exactly what *The Cognitive Behavioral Workbook for Menopause* is designed to provide. This workbook makes clear that there are a wide range of approaches to treatment, and while this book steps forward with the strengths of a cognitive behavioral approach to coping, it does so while also discussing the benefits of a range of alternative therapies. Hormone replacement, acupuncture, and natural therapeutics, like red clover, black cohosh, omega-3 fatty acids, and Saint-John's-wort, all get their due. Likewise, this workbook does not assume that one treatment size fits all. Women will differ in which symptoms are most pronounced during any one phase of the menopausal transition, and likewise, different elements of this workbook, treatments, or combinations of treatment may be most relevant for any given phase. To meet this variability, women need to be educated about menopause, its symptoms, and the stages of the menopausal transition. This workbook offers information and interventions grounded in the latest scientific studies.

The workbook is written by a team of experts, bringing you perspectives from women's health, clinical psychiatry, and clinical and health psychology. Likewise, their clinical work includes pharmacologic as well as the cognitive behavioral interventions that form the core of this book. The result is readers are assured to get expert information that is informed by the latest scientific findings and is complemented by case examples providing a personal perspective on symptoms and coping.

As for the clinical content of this book, I can't express how pleased I am that this workbook makes cognitive behavioral interventions so readily available. Cognitive behavioral therapy offers individuals with a wide range of disorders some of the best outcomes in psychiatry. It is a focused, practical, and collaborative approach that takes a woman from her current experience of symptoms and steps forward with a framework for greater coping. Accordingly, for the varied mood and somatic symptoms of the menopausal transition, a cognitive behavioral approach provides a good fit for the changing targets of distress that define this time of vulnerability. As the authors discuss, any one chapter may have greater or less interest, depending on the phase of menopausal transition and the symptoms that are most prominent in a woman's life at that time. Accordingly, the importance of individual chapters of this book will change over time, as readers match the information provided to their specific needs.

The workbook format ensures that women don't just learn about treatment abstractly but are engaged in the practice of change that makes a difference. So, whether it is learning a more mindful approach to hot flashes, reducing their likelihood of occurrence, or keeping a fresh shirt handy for an especially drenching episode, women will learn a toolbox of approaches for keeping mood and life goals on track during this vulnerable time.

> —Michael W. Otto, PhD
> Professor of Psychology, Boston University
> Author of *Living with Bipolar Disorder*
> and *Exercise for Mood and Anxiety:*
> *Proven Strategies for Overcoming*
> *Depression and Enhancing Well-Being*

Acknowledgments

My understanding of the cognitive behavioral model began early on in my training, in graduate classes, workshops, and readings from cognitive experts. However, it was not until I engaged in my first clinical practicum experience, treating patients with anxiety disorders, that I witnessed just how powerful this theory was when put into practice. People's lives significantly changed as a result of participating in CBT, and being in a position to facilitate this change motivated me to specialize in this area. I feel that it is important to acknowledge the mentors who helped me develop and hone my skills as a cognitive behavioral therapist, including Dr. R. McCabe, Dr. M. Antony, Dr. P. Bieling, Dr. T. Hadjistavropoulos, Dr. N. Rector, and Dr. M. Lau. Thank you for your guidance, challenges, and patience. You have helped me think outside the box in terms of implementing traditional CBT treatment protocols, to hopefully reach many more individuals experiencing distress.

—S. M. G.

We would like to acknowledge and express our gratitude to the following individuals who shared their menopausal experiences by responding to our survey: Barbara Hammond, Sharon Lloyd, Gail McCabe, Edna Toth, Teresa Vall, Ghislaine Yergeau, and Elaine Green. Also important to acknowledge are the participants in the CBT group for menopausal symptoms, whose experiences and responses to treatment helped shape the content of this book.

We would like to thank the editors and staff at New Harbinger Publications, especially Melissa Kirk, for their guidance and valuable feedback while writing this book. We are also grateful to Rachel Strimas for taking the time to read and provide helpful feedback and comments on our manuscript. Finally, we would like to acknowledge and deeply thank our families for their support and understanding during the writing of this book.

—S. M. G., R. E. M., & C. N. S.

Introduction

Out of the blue, the heat came upon me and the sweat started rolling down my face. I tried to dab it away and focus on the dinner conversation. My hair started to become damp and I felt like I had run a marathon. I wondered what was going on with my body!

When I entered menopause, I realized that I was embarking on a different stage in my life. I was not sure how I felt about it. I started to have thoughts about what it meant and what my purpose in life was. I felt a sense of loss that I struggled to understand.

My relationship with my husband became strained as I found sexual intimacy difficult due to the changes that were happening in my body related to menopause. I felt like I was drying up, and intercourse became increasingly painful.

I have always been a stable and upbeat person, but since approaching menopause, I have noticed that my mood is all over the place. I am irritable with my family and find that I am acting more edgy than ever.

It is hard to remember the last time I had a full night's sleep since I have been going through menopause. My mind is busy all night, and I find myself worrying about all sorts of things that do not seem as important in the morning.

Every woman's experience of menopause is different. Unlike a disorder or disease, menopause is a natural transition that all women go through in their lives. Nevertheless, this transition can be accompanied by unpleasant symptoms that can really have a negative impact on your daily functioning and overall quality of life.

Symptoms during menopause vary from woman to woman, just as menstrual cycles or pregnancy and postpartum periods do. Some women experience a number of unpleasant symptoms associated with their menstrual cycle, such as mood swings and cramping, while other women experience none at all. For most women, pregnancy and the postpartum period are quite often joyful, but some women struggle with mood swings, extreme exhaustion, or even depression. Similarly, menopausal symptoms affect everyone differently in terms of their severity and the extent to which they interfere with day-to-day functioning and lifestyle.

HOW THIS BOOK CAN HELP

Given that you are reading this book, we can assume that your life has been negatively affected by the menopausal symptoms you are experiencing. This book is for any woman who is going through menopause, whether you are going through menopause naturally, as a result of aging, or because of a *hysterectomy* and *oophorectomy* (the surgical removal of the uterus and ovaries). We designed this workbook to treat your menopausal symptoms or to complement other treatments that you may currently be receiving. The strategies in this book were developed to address a real gap that we saw in the available treatment options. Many women who came to our clinic were having their lives greatly disrupted by menopausal symptoms, yet the available treatments, such as hormonal replacement therapy (HRT), antidepressants, or herbal medications, were either insufficient or not recommended for them. Like these women, you may be in one of the following situations:

- Current medical treatments are not recommended for you, because you are at a higher risk for various health problems, such as breast cancer.

- You are receiving treatment but are not fully satisfied with it, because of either your response to the treatment or the side effects caused by it.

- You are experiencing some degree of impairment in functioning or an unmanageable level of symptom severity despite receiving one or more treatments.

- Current treatments are working for you, but you would prefer to use self-management techniques and strategies to decrease the severity of your symptoms rather than rely on so many medications and supplements.

If you find that you can relate to any of these scenarios, then this book is for you!

HOW THIS PROGRAM WORKS

This book is designed to help you with the symptoms you may be experiencing and struggling with right now. Part 1 will help you learn more about the menopausal transition: what is involved, including the types of symptoms you may be experiencing and why you are experiencing them. Part 1 also covers how various treatments can help you cope with what you are going through and will help you plan how to use this book's approach to address your most distressing symptoms.

In part 2, you will want to focus on the chapters that specifically address the symptoms you are struggling with. For example, if sleep difficulty is your most prominent symptom, you will go straight to chapter

8. If hot flashes are your biggest problem, then you will start with chapter 5 instead. The goal is to give you some immediate relief from your most distressing symptoms. If you are experiencing a number of difficult symptoms, we recommend that you focus first on the symptom that is most distressing or is interfering the most in your life. Once you have addressed that symptom, you can move on to the next problematic symptom on your list. The treatment approach that this book offers is called *cognitive behavioral therapy,* or CBT.

COGNITIVE BEHAVIORAL THERAPY

Cognitive behavioral therapy is a psychological treatment approach that has been shown to be highly effective for addressing the emotional symptoms of anxiety and depression, as well as a range of health issues including chronic pain and menopausal symptoms. CBT focuses on understanding how your thoughts, physical symptoms, and behaviors interact to cause you distress. Using CBT, you will learn specific strategies to reduce unhelpful thought patterns and to improve your behavioral responses to uncomfortable symptoms and stressors.

Maximizing the Benefits of This Approach

To experience the maximum benefits from this approach, you will need to make yourself and CBT a top priority. How can you make time in your busy life to read this book, learn the strategies, and practice them? You will need to set aside time each day with the goal of working your way through this book. The more time you devote to practicing the strategies introduced here, the greater benefit you will experience in your quality of life. It may help to set aside a specific time in your schedule to work on this every day, such as at your lunch break or before bedtime. It can also be helpful to go through this process with someone else. If you have a friend who is also going through the menopausal transition or early menopausal years and is looking to gain relief from her symptoms, you can work on strategies together and provide mutual support and encouragement. Alternatively, checking in regularly with a health care provider can also provide support and motivation.

HOW THIS BOOK CAME ABOUT

In 2006, the three of us met to discuss ideas for a collaborative research project that would capture our mutual interests and draw on our different areas of expertise: health psychology and CBT (Sheryl Green), anxiety and CBT (Randi McCabe), and psychiatry, women's health, and menopause (Claudio Soares). The topic of menopausal treatment came up as we considered both the lack of nonmedicinal options for women experiencing menopause and the number of symptoms associated with the menopausal transition, such as sleep difficulties, anxiety, and depression, that have been successfully treated through psychological means on their own.

After developing a treatment protocol based on CBT strategies, we received a small grant to facilitate a pilot study to determine the effectiveness of this treatment for menopausal symptoms. The findings from this pilot study demonstrated that the treatment was successful both in reducing the number of debilitating symptoms that can occur as a result of menopause and in improving overall quality of life (Green et al. 2010). The treatment was well received by participants, who reported high levels of satisfaction.

The idea for this book came toward the tail end of the pilot study, as we wanted to reach as many women as possible with a potential alternative or complementary treatment for their menopausal symptoms. We also wanted to provide our treatment protocol in a workbook form that could be used by both women going through menopause and care providers. Although a number of books address menopausal symptoms, we found the need for a workbook that would allow the user to learn and implement CBT strategies in an interactive way and with an approach tailored to her specific needs.

PART 1

Menopause, Its Symptoms, and Your Treatment Options

CHAPTER 1

Learning about Menopause

What is happening to my body?

What are the changes occurring in my body that lead into the menopausal transition?

What stage of the menopausal transition am I experiencing right now?

What are the symptoms that I may experience during menopause?

It is important to understand what exactly is happening to your body as you go through the menopausal transition and beyond. As with any difficulty or challenge, understanding what's happening to you can help you cope. This chapter provides an overview of the physiological process of menopause. The more you learn about the changes your body is going through, the better positioned you will be to strategically manage your symptoms.

FACTS AND PHYSIOLOGY

To understand menopause and its common symptoms, a good starting point is to look at the changes that occur during the transition from childhood through puberty. Puberty marks the time when significant hormonal changes first begin in your life, signifying the commencement of your reproductive years. Similarly, with the start of menopause, another significant hormonal shift takes place, associated this time with the end of your reproductive years.

Puberty and the Reproductive Years

Puberty typically occurs in girls at twelve to fourteen years of age, when they begin to develop breasts and show other signs of sexual maturation. A number of associated hormonal changes also trigger the ability to reproduce, which is marked by the start of menstruation. An increase in the brain of the luteinizing hormone (LH) and the follicle-stimulating hormone (FSH) triggers the ovaries to produce the sex hormones estrogen and progesterone. Both estrogen and progesterone serve a number of major functions, and key among them is activation of the menstrual cycle.

The average menstrual cycle is twenty-eight days in duration. A cycle consists of three main phases:

FOLLICULAR PHASE

The follicular phase includes the first day of menstruation, or your period, up to ovulation. This is roughly day one to day fourteen of your cycle. During this phase, estrogen levels gradually increase, causing the lining of the uterus to thicken in preparation for a potential pregnancy and causing follicles to begin developing within the ovaries. One or two of these follicles becomes dominant, or destined for ovulation, while the rest die.

OVULATION

During ovulation, there is a sharp rise in LH and FSH levels, and the dominant follicles release an egg. The typical length of this phase is twenty-four to forty-eight hours. It is during this phase that fertilization can take place.

LUTEAL PHASE

During the luteal phase, large amounts of progesterone are produced, which causes changes in the uterine lining, preparing it for implantation of a fertilized egg (embryo) and pregnancy. If no eggs are fertilized or there is no implantation, the levels of both estrogen and progesterone drop sharply, and the lining of the uterus is shed through menstruation, which marks the start of a new reproductive cycle. The luteal phase lasts twelve to sixteen days.

This twenty-eight-day cyclical process typically continues through your lifetime from the onset of puberty with your first menstruation (also called *menarche*) until the menopausal transition begins. Figure 1.1 shows how different hormone levels typically rise and fall during the twenty-eight-day cycle.

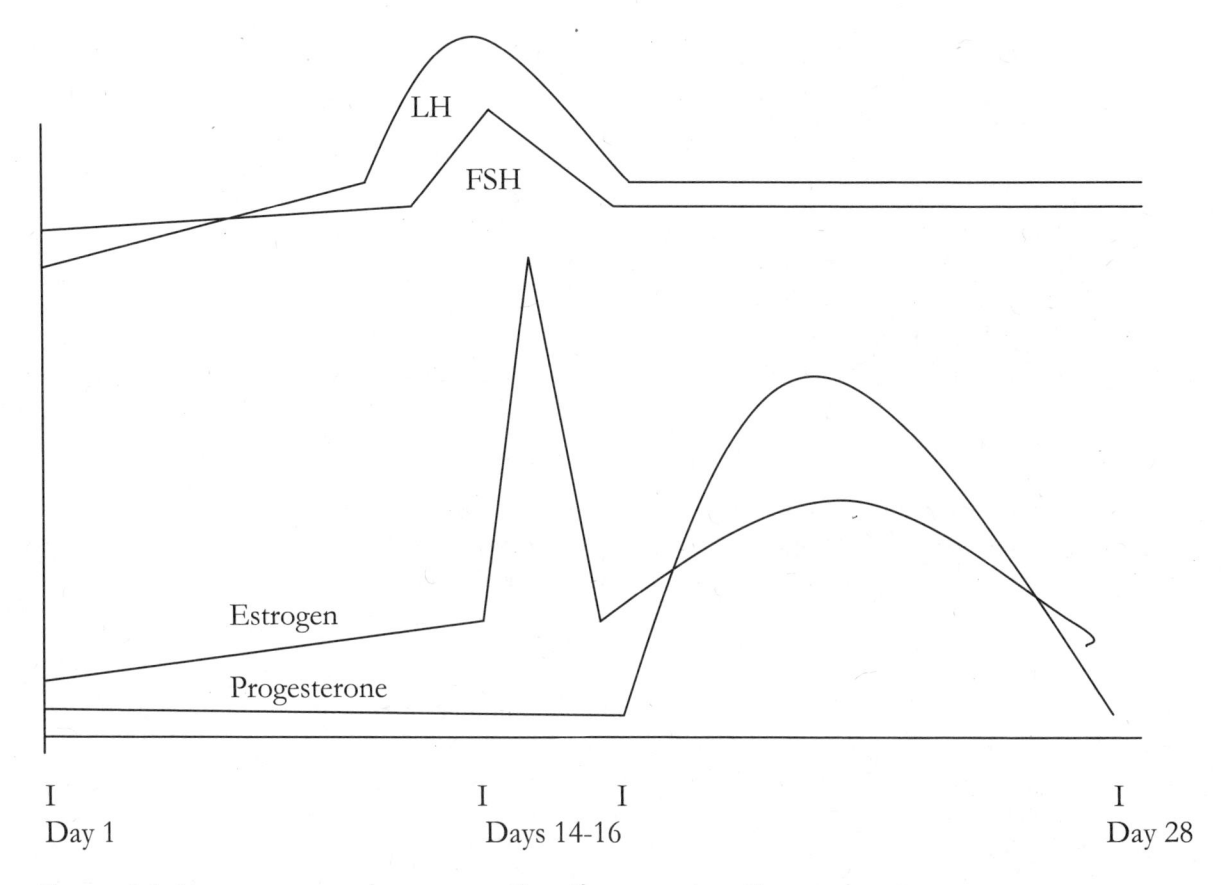

Figure 1.1: Hormone graph representing the menstruation cycle

It may help to consider that the changing hormone levels depicted in figure 1—and any negative symptoms you may associate with menstruation—are a routine fact of life for most women from around age twelve to fourteen through their late forties. The new symptoms that you are experiencing at this point in your life are associated with the ending of this cyclical process.

Menopause Timeline

The *menopausal transition* is defined as the time preceding the final menstrual period when variability in the menstrual cycle usually increases (WHO Scientific Group 1996). Menopause is recognized to have occurred after twelve months following the final menstrual period (Soules et al. 2001). The menopausal transition and menopause occur naturally in four defined stages: early perimenopause, late perimenopause, early postmenopause, and late postmenopause. As you read about each stage below, you may want to consider where you are in the process.

PERIMENOPAUSE AND EARLY PERIMENOPAUSE

Perimenopause is defined as the phase of time immediately preceding the final menstrual period in your life and the first twelve months after your final menstrual period (WHO Scientific Group 1996). This phase generally begins at forty-seven or forty-eight years of age and lasts for an average of four years. This time in a woman's life marks the dynamic progression from a state of routine hormonal changes to cessation of menses as a consequence of the ovaries ceasing to function.

The *early perimenopause* stage is marked by an increase in your FSH levels and slight variations in your menstrual cycle. This might occur sooner than you think (some women enter this stage in their early forties). Changes in your menstrual cycle at this point can be very subtle. For example, your periods may be longer or shorter than usual or may be more or less frequent. During this stage, you might also start to notice some common menopausal symptoms, such as hot flashes and night sweats, difficulties in sexual functioning, or sleep complaints, although these symptoms are usually more pronounced during later stages. As you enter this stage, you may find that you are more susceptible to moodiness, depression, or anxiety.

LATE PERIMENOPAUSE

Late perimenopause begins when you have missed at least two consecutive menstrual cycles, which means that your menstrual cycle is becoming more erratic. Your FSH levels continue to increase, and you may start to notice that the symptoms that developed earlier have now become more common or more intense.

MENOPAUSE AND EARLY POSTMENOPAUSE

Menopause is defined by twelve consecutive months without menstrual cycles (in the absence of pregnancy or other causes). After that, you are officially in *early postmenopause*, a stage that starts twelve months after your final period and lasts for no more than four years. During this time, your FSH levels increase, and you may continue to experience intense symptoms, especially hot flashes, sexual dysfunction, and sleep disruption.

LATE POSTMENOPAUSE

The final stage begins five years after your final menstrual period. Symptoms are not typically experienced any longer, although some women have reportedly experienced hot flashes and night sweats for as long as twelve years after their final menstrual period. Your FSH levels will have reached their peak, and your ovaries' production of estrogen will significantly decline.

Surgical Menopause

Menopause can also be induced by surgery through the removal of the uterus or the ovaries. If you had a hysterectomy earlier in your life (for example, in your thirties), but you still have your ovaries, you may experience menopause-related symptoms much later on due to changes in your hormone levels, though your periods will have stopped when you had the surgery. Either surgery can bring on menopausal symptoms.

Learning about Menopause

> ## Where Are You on the Menopausal Timeline?
>
> Answer the following questions to determine where you are on the menopausal timeline:
>
> 1. Are you experiencing subtle changes in your menstrual cycles? Are they getting heavier/lighter, shorter/longer?
>
> 2. Have you skipped menstruation a few times over the past year but still had most of your cycles?
>
> 3. Are you having intense hot flashes or night sweats, or broken sleep?
>
> 4. Are you skipping menstrual cycles more often (for example, going without menses for a few months in a row but still having periods from time to time)?
>
> 5. Did you have your last menstrual period more than a year ago without any obvious reasons, such as surgery, pregnancy, or hormonal treatments?
>
> If you answered yes to 1 and/or 2, you are probably in early perimenopause.
>
> If you answered yes to 3 and 4, you are probably in late perimenopause.
>
> If you answered yes to 5, you are probably in early postmenopause (within the first five years).

HOW HORMONAL CHANGES AFFECT YOU

Most women experience one or more physical and emotional discomforts during the menopausal transition. These discomforts are often related to the hormonal changes that your body is going through.

The Role of Estrogen

Estrogen plays an important role in both your psychological and your physical well-being. Psychologically, major changes or fluctuations in your estrogen levels and other sex hormones (such as testosterone) have a significant impact on your mood, sleep, and sexual drive, or libido. Therefore, when your ovarian production of estrogen starts to fluctuate—sometimes in a chaotic way—many of your body systems are affected. This is why women may experience any among a number of different psychological and physical symptoms during the menopausal transition: hot flashes and night sweats, sleep disturbances, changes in mood, and changes in sexual functioning, such as decreased libido and vaginal dryness. Any of these symptoms can affect your quality of life and your overall functioning.

Recent studies show that, for some women, the menopausal transition is a period of heightened risk for depression and anxiety, either as a new onset or a recurrent episode (Cohen et al. 2006). Depression in midlife women may be a complex, multifaceted phenomenon. Several factors may contribute to depression at this point in a woman's life, including medical conditions, lifestyle, and sleep changes, but there are certain known risk factors. African-American women are at higher risk for depression whereas Asian-Americans are at lower risk; a family history of depression, a history of postpartum blues or depression, and stressful life events also increase the risk for depression (Cohen et al. 2006; Bromberger and Kravitz 2011).

More recently, researchers have proposed a *timing theory* or a *window of vulnerability* for depression and other complaints during the menopausal transition. This vulnerability seems to be associated with intense fluctuations in sex hormones, particularly estrogen levels. An interesting fact is that it is the fluctuation itself, rather than low levels or deficiency of estrogen, which seems to increase the risk. The greater the fluctuations in sex hormones over the transition, the greater the risk for depression, probably because of the cross talk between estrogen and other neurotransmitters in your brain that regulate mood and behavior (Soares 2010; Lokuge et al. 2011).

Physically, estrogen is involved in the functioning of your urinary tract, skin, vaginal tissues, bones, heart, and blood vessels, and the health of your gums, teeth, and eyes. In addition, changes in metabolism occurring at the same time as menopause may lead to an increased risk for cardiovascular disease (Teede 2007).

Other Life Factors

The transition to menopause is often accompanied by other life changes associated with growing older. For instance, your adult children may be leaving home, you may be retiring early, or you may have taken on some new roles, such as becoming a grandparent or a caregiver to aging parents. These circumstances can also affect your mood and self-esteem. Any change, even a positive one, can add stress to your life. Such stress may exacerbate menopausal symptoms as well as challenge your coping abilities.

COMMON MENOPAUSAL SYMPTOMS

You likely have had firsthand experience with some menopausal symptoms, given that you are reading this book. This section will review each of the symptoms commonly associated with the menopausal transition. As you read about them, you may want to reflect on which symptoms you've experienced and what impact they've had on you. The next chapter will help you look at each of your symptoms in more detail.

Vasomotor Symptoms

"The hot flashes just come out of the blue, making it difficult to interact with people at work and socialize during my time off without becoming embarrassed that others have noticed how hot and sweaty I have become."

Vasomotor symptoms are more commonly known as hot flashes and night sweats. These are spontaneous episodes of warmth and/or sweating that you usually feel on your chest, neck, and face. Hot flashes occur when the blood vessels that are close to your skin suddenly dilate and open. Studies have shown that vasomotor symptoms reflect a dysregulation of your core body temperature, a complex and delicate system involving particular areas of your brain (such as the hypothalamus) and sensors throughout your body (Freedman 2005). Fluctuations in your levels of estrogen and of the neurotransmitters serotonin and norepinephrine result in hot flashes, as these changes influence your body's temperature regulation center.

Sleep Disturbance

"The night sweats that I get disrupt my sleep tremendously, as I often have to get up and change my soaking-wet pajamas."

Many women report sleep disruption during menopause. Night sweats can disrupt your sleep and affect both the amount and the quality of sleep you get. For instance, when a night sweat wakes you up, you may have to get out of bed to change your clothes and then find it difficult to get back to sleep. If this happens on a regular basis, you may discover that lack of sleep and sleep disruption affect your functioning during the day. It is important to note that disrupted sleep may also occur in the absence of night sweats; significant weight changes, sleep apnea, anxiety, and poor sleep hygiene can affect sleep and sometimes require further investigation.

Mood/Depression

"Lately, I get saddened whenever I hear about the child of a friend or colleague who has recently graduated from university, gotten married, or has had a child of their own, as these are experiences I will never have."

During perimenopause and menopause, it is not uncommon to experience episodes of sadness. A decline in estrogen can affect your mental and emotional health, and a connection between depression and menopause has been found (Cohen et al. 2006). However, in addition to the hormonal link to depression, a number of other things may be risk factors for depression, including stressful events in your life, heredity, and seasonal changes.

If you have made the decision not to have children, you may also experience feelings of sadness, loss, and regret during this time, as menopause marks the end of your ability to conceive. You may have also noticed yourself being more irritable, as well as sudden shifts in your mood. You may feel that your moods are all over the place and that you can suddenly shift from feeling okay and positive to feeling down and negative.

Urogenital Problems and Sexual Concerns

"My husband and I both continue to be interested in having sex, but the vaginal dryness that I experience makes it very painful and, ultimately, not very enjoyable."

Vaginal dryness and atrophy (thinning of the wall of the vagina) result from reduced local and systemic estrogen levels and frequently occur during menopause. Painful intercourse due to vaginal dryness can make it hard for you to engage in or enjoy sex. Further, a lower libido can result during menopause as a consequence both of hormone imbalance and of seeing yourself as unattractive and undesirable because of your other symptoms, such as hot flashes.

During menopause, many women also experience stress or urge incontinence. Stress incontinence is an involuntary loss of urine during a physical activity, such as coughing, sneezing, or laughing, or while exercising. It is often seen in women who have had multiple pregnancies and vaginal childbirths. Aging and obesity increase the risk for stress incontinence associated with a depletion of estrogen. Urge incontinence is a strong, sudden need to urinate at day or nighttime, leading to some leakage or involuntary loss of urine. Urge incontinence may occur in anyone at any age but is more common in women with a depletion of estrogen and in the elderly. Losing control of your bladder can have a devastating impact, making such everyday activities as laughing or walking possible triggers for urinary incontinence. You may also find you need to urinate more often; a frequent urge to empty your bladder may have a negative effect on your daily quality of life or disrupt your sleep when it occurs at night.

Anxiety

"Last night I walked into the supermarket and out of the blue began to feel very hot, short of breath, and my heart began to race. I wasn't sure whether this was the start of a hot flash or just my anxiety. I started to become anxious that I could not catch my breath and that others could see that there was something wrong with me. My symptoms increased until I was experiencing a full-blown panic attack."

A rapid drop in your estrogen levels may increase your experience of anxiety. You may also experience anxiety when a hot flash is coming on if you misread the physical symptoms as a sign that something is seriously wrong with you. If so, you may find that your physical symptoms escalate into more intense anxiety or even turn into a panic attack.

It is also not uncommon for women in menopause to have trouble differentiating between a hot flash and an anxiety attack, because these two conditions can cause similar feelings: sudden, unexpected waves of physical discomfort that are frequently accompanied by intense sweating and heat dissipation, heart palpitation, and shortness of breath. Even if you have no trouble recognizing a hot flash for what it is, the physical discomforts associated with it quite often provoke awkward situations in social settings or in the workplace, and you may find yourself changing your daily routine to avoid facing these symptoms in public.

Anxiety can take many different forms. Some people notice an overall increase in their level of anxiety whereas others report more intense episodes of anxiety. If you suffer from anxiety, you may find yourself avoiding parties or other social gatherings that you associate with feeling uncomfortable.

IDENTIFYING YOUR SYMPTOMS

As you can see, the menopausal transition has been linked to a wide range of both physical and emotional symptoms and can make you vulnerable to anxiety and depression. Again, every woman reacts differently to the symptoms that she experiences, and your experience of this time of life will be unique.

It is a good idea to check with your doctor to confirm that the symptoms you are experiencing are primarily related to menopause and to be sure that you don't have any other conditions or illnesses in need of treatment. Also, if you are experiencing significant symptoms of depression or anxiety, we recommend scheduling a visit with your doctor to learn about additional treatment options that may be available to you. You want to ask your doctor the following:

- Are the symptoms you are experiencing primarily related to menopause?

- Are your symptoms related to a condition or illness unrelated to menopause that is in need of medical assessment and treatment?

- If you are having significant symptoms of depression or anxiety, are there additional treatment options available, such as medical treatment or cognitive behavioral therapy with a mental health professional?

This chapter has given you an overview of what occurs during menopause and the symptoms commonly connected with it. Chapter 2 will help you examine the symptoms you are experiencing and the impact they're having on your day-to-day functioning and overall lifestyle.

SUMMING IT ALL UP

- Puberty marks the start of your menstruation cycles, which result in production of follicle-stimulating hormone and luteinizing hormone, as well as the sex hormones estrogen and progesterone. Reproduction becomes possible at this time.

- Menopause can occur either naturally or surgically. If occurring naturally, it has four stages: early perimenopause, late perimenopause, early postmenopause, and late postmenopause.

- The menopausal transition is often referred to as a window of vulnerability. As your estrogen production reduces or fluctuates widely, you may experience a number of unpleasant symptoms, including hot flashes and night sweats, sleep disruption, mood and anxiety symptoms, urogenital problems, and changes in sexual drive, or libido.

- Not all women experience significant menopausal symptoms; symptoms and their impact differ from woman to woman.

- You may want to schedule a visit with your doctor to confirm that the symptoms you are experiencing are primarily related to menopause and to identify any additional treatments that may be available to you, particularly if you are experiencing significant levels of anxiety or depression.

CHAPTER 2

Recognizing Your Symptoms

How is the menopausal transition affecting me?

What symptoms am I experiencing?

How much are my symptoms bothering me and interfering with my lifestyle?

Increasing Your Self-Awareness

The first step is to reflect on your experience and ask yourself what menopausal symptoms you are experiencing. For example, sleep disturbance is often a problem during the menopausal transition, and it may be an issue for you. If you decide that it is, we encourage you to reflect on your experience further to determine if the problem is that you're getting less sleep than usual or, alternatively, you're getting enough sleep but you frequently wake up during the night. The latter would be affecting the quality of your sleep. The next step would be to try to figure out why your sleep is broken.

You might be aware that you are having problems with your sleep but have not really taken the time to reflect on what is contributing to this problem. Perhaps your sleep is broken due to overheating caused by night sweats or the disruption of getting up and changing your clothes. Urinary incontinence might be the culprit, or you may find it hard to shut down your mind due to anxious thoughts.

The greater your awareness of how menopausal symptoms affect you, the better you can address them. There are many strategies that could be employed with sleep disruption, for example, but you will want to choose your approach based on knowledge of the cause. We want you to become the expert on your own condition so that you can monitor the effectiveness of various treatment strategies on your menopausal symptoms over time.

THE FACES OF MENOPAUSE

Each woman's experience of menopause is different. One woman may have multiple symptoms that have a minimal impact on her life, whereas another woman might report only one symptom, but that symptom may cause her significant difficulty. The following four stories illustrate how every woman's experience is unique:

■ *Jane*

Age: fifty-five

Menopausal stage: early postmenopause

Main symptom: hot flashes

Jane is a married mother of one. She works full time as a caregiver to seniors. Jane started experiencing menopausal symptoms when she was fifty-two, and mainly she complained of hot flashes. When the hot flashes first started, she noticed that she could predict, at times, that they would occur when she was very busy at work. However, when Jane entered the early postmenopause phase, she noticed that the sweating had gone into overdrive. She would be sitting at a dinner party and, out of nowhere, start sweating so much that she felt she looked as if she'd just run a marathon.

Jane found this symptom distressing on many levels. She disliked being unable to predict when it would happen. She found it embarrassing, especially at work meetings and social events. Hot flashes were affecting her ability to concentrate and socialize with friends and family. She felt uncomfortable. Her clothes would become soaked, and she had to carry around a change of clothing, just in case she needed it.

Jane had always been confident and self-assured, but she found the unexpected sweating episodes left her feeling exposed and vulnerable. She felt that her hot flashes were taking over her life and wanted to do something to change this.

■ *Catherine*

Age: fifty

Menopausal stage: late perimenopause

Main symptom: depression

Catherine is a schoolteacher who lives alone and does not have any children. Now in late perimenopause, she is experiencing a depressed mood and a loss of energy.

Catherine used to put a lot of time and effort into her career. She enjoyed it and was successful. Over the years, she received a number of teaching awards. Now Catherine finds less enjoyment in work than formerly and feels that she's just putting in her time before retiring from teaching.

Until recently, Catherine was also very social, but now she finds herself often declining invitations to do things with friends and family. She has become rather withdrawn and isolated. With the cessation of her periods, she feels sadder than she used to feel when reflecting on her decision to remain single and childless. She finds herself dwelling on how she might be alone and unhappy for years to come. With the onset of menopause, Catherine is questioning her role and the meaning of her life.

■ *Gloria*

Age: fifty-six

Menopausal stage: early postmenopause

Main symptom: sleep disruption

Gloria is a married homemaker with three stepchildren. Her main complaint is sleep disruption. She also feels sad much of the time, but she thinks that she's sad mostly because she's not sleeping. She believes that she would feel better if only she could get a good night's sleep.

Gloria describes experiencing night sweats that wake her up. Typically, she gets up and changes from soaked pajamas into something dry, disrupting her partner's sleep in the process. Once awake, Gloria finds it difficult to get back to sleep, as her mind is then occupied by anxious thoughts about everything that has to be done over the coming week. As a result, she loses more sleep and starts the next day feeling drained and low on coping resources.

■ *Ellen*

Age: forty-nine

Menopausal stage: late perimenopause

Main symptom: anxiety

Ellen works full time as a cashier and is a married mother of two adult children. Ellen has begun to have hot flashes where she experiences intense waves of heat on her chest, neck, and face. She has also noticed other physical sensations, such as sweating, shortness of breath, and a racing heart. The physical sensations that Ellen experiences while having a hot flash are very similar to the sensations that she experienced during an earlier period in her life when she suffered from panic attacks. Now Ellen has started to become confused as to whether she is having a hot flash or a panic attack.

In previous panic attacks, Ellen feared that she might faint. Now her fear is that she might have another panic attack, and she has begun worrying about when the next one will arrive. When she noticed that she was beginning to avoid driving and going to the grocery store because she was afraid of having a panic attack in public, Ellen realized that she needed to get some help.

These four stories illustrate some of the symptoms that women experience during menopause and the effect they can have. Perhaps you can relate to one or more of these women's experiences. To examine your experience of menopause more closely, take some time to complete the following menopause symptom checklist. This checklist identifies the most common symptoms associated with the menopausal transition.

Menopause Symptom Checklist

For each of the following menopausal symptoms that you recognize yourself as having, describe your experience of the symptom in the space provided. If you've noticed another change that you suspect is a symptom but is not listed below, you can describe it at the end of the list. Use the heading "other."

Vasomotor symptoms (hot flashes, night sweats)
_____

Sleep disturbance (frequent wakening, insomnia)
_____

Mood changes/depression (mood swings, low mood, sad mood, lack of interest, lack of pleasure, social withdrawal, negative thoughts about yourself or others, hopelessness, lack of energy)
_____

Urogenital problems (urinary incontinence, vaginal dryness, atrophy)
_____

Sexual concerns (lack of libido or sexual drive, vaginal dryness)
_____

Anxiety (panic attacks, worries, increased fear and arousal, avoidance)
_____

Other
_____

Other
_____

   Now you should have a better idea of which menopausal symptoms are an issue for you and how you experience them. The next exercise will help you look at how going through menopause is affecting your life more generally.

How Has Menopause Affected Your Life?

Take a few minutes now to assess the impact of your symptoms on your life. Consider how going through menopause is affecting your daily life and reflect on how this phase of life may have affected your view of yourself and your own personal meaning. Use the questions below to guide your reflections, and write down your thoughts in the space provided.

1. How has menopause affected your quality of life and day-to-day functioning?

   _____
   _____
   _____
   _____
   _____

2. How has menopause affected your view of yourself?

   _____
   _____
   _____
   _____
   _____

3. How has menopause affected your view of life and your future?

   _____
   _____
   _____
   _____
   _____

You may find that some of the symptoms you are experiencing are a daily nuisance. Your symptoms may have had a negative effect on your work and social life, your enjoyment of leisure activities, and the quality of your relationships. You may have also found that the menopause transition has been accompanied by changes in how you feel about yourself and your future. Many women find themselves questioning the meaning of their lives, reevaluating decisions that they have made, or looking at the aging process and the future from a new vantage point. One woman in late menopause commented that she had stopped "just living" and had started thinking about her life in terms of the years she had remaining. In later chapters, you will learn some strategies to tackle your symptoms and help you look at the future with a healthy sense of purpose.

You also may not be aware of how menopausal symptoms are contributing to your difficulties. To help you become more aware of all your symptoms and how they are affecting your life, you may want to keep a symptom diary. Try using the following diary to record any changes or symptoms you notice over the next week. Record the symptom as soon as you can after it occurs so that you will remember the details. If that's not possible, then set aside some time each day to write in your diary.

You may want to record your symptoms for an additional week to capture any symptoms that you experience less frequently. If you think you'll want to reuse this worksheet, you can make photocopies before filling it in.

Weekly Menopause Symptom Diary

Complete this worksheet over the next week, recording any symptoms you notice each day. Identify and describe any hot flashes, night sweats, sleep disturbance, stress or urge incontinence, sexual concerns, mood changes/depression, anxiety, or other symptoms you experience. Note the context in which they occur: whom you were with, what you were doing, where you were, and when this symptom happened. Also note the impact on you: what effect the symptom had on how you were thinking, feeling, and behaving. The diary includes an example.

Date	Symptom and Description	Situation/Context	Impact
Example:	*Hot flash: flushed face, sweating through my shirt, feeling very uncomfortable, sweat dripping down my face, had to keep wiping it away*	*In a meeting at work*	*Had difficulty concentrating on what I was saying. I was concerned that people would notice and wonder what was going on with me. I felt very embarrassed.*
Day 1			
Day 2			
Day 3			
Day 4			
Day 5			
Day 6			
Day 7			

Reflecting on What You've Learned

Now take a moment to step back and see what you have learned. Were there any symptoms you recorded that you had not been aware of previously? Do you notice any patterns in terms of context? Do you notice any effects on your life that you had not noticed before? This information is important. It will be useful material to work with later when you will choose strategies for managing your symptoms and reducing their impact on your life. If you find that you experienced symptoms that you did not record on the menopause symptom checklist, please update the list.

Now that you have recorded your symptoms, the next step is to prioritize them in terms of their severity and negative impact on your life. This will help you decide which symptom to tackle first.

Symptom Rating Form

Record every symptom that you experience and rate each symptom in terms of its severity and its interference in your life. Use the following two scales of 0 to 100 as a guide as you rate each symptom:

Severity/Intensity

0	10	20	30	40	50	60	70	80	90	100
not at all severe			mildly severe			moderately severe			most severe	

Interference/Impact

0	10	20	30	40	50	60	70	80	90	100
not at all interfering			mildly interfering			moderately interfering			most interfering	

First rate the symptom's severity (intensity), where 0 is not at all severe and 100 is the most severe. Then rate the symptom's interference (impact), where 0 is no interference and 100 is the greatest interference.

Symptom Description	Severity/ Intensity 0–100	Interference/ Impact 0–100
Example: *hot flashes*	65	85
1.		
2.		
3.		
4.		
5.		
6.		
7.		
8.		

Your symptom rating form may list many symptoms or only one symptom. You may discover that your symptoms vary greatly in severity and impact, or you may find that your symptoms are quite comparable in terms of how intense they are or how much they interfere with your life. This symptom rating form will guide you and help direct your energy in part 2 as you begin to tackle your symptoms. We recommend focusing your efforts first on the symptom that is most distressing. If you find that some of your symptoms are equal in their intensity and impact, then you may choose whichever you prefer to focus on first. You can easily refer back to the list whenever you are ready to tackle the next symptom.

SUMMING IT ALL UP

- The first step in tackling your menopausal symptoms is to increase your awareness of the symptoms you are experiencing.

- Monitoring your symptoms using the weekly menopause symptom diary allows you to evaluate the intensity of your symptoms and the degree to which they are having a negative effect on your life.

- Prioritizing your symptoms in terms of their severity and impact allows you to determine where you will focus your symptom management efforts first.

CHAPTER 3

Choosing among the Treatment Options

What do I need to know about hormone therapy?

Are other medication options available?

What are some alternative treatment options?

You may be looking for the best strategies to cope with the changes your body is going through during this time in your life. This chapter is all about options. The bad news is that there is no silver bullet or perfect solution for the array of symptoms that you may be experiencing. The good news is that choosing how to focus your treatment and ultimately achieve your goals might be easier than you think. It's time to get started.

HORMONE THERAPY

Previous chapters have discussed the important contribution of hormonal changes to most of your menopausal symptoms. With that in mind, the following question almost always comes up: if hormonal changes can cause these symptoms, could hormone therapy help alleviate them?

For many decades, the use of hormone therapy for menopausal symptoms—traditionally called *hormone replacement therapy* (HRT)—was widely accepted and considered to be practically a silver bullet. The discussion about the potential risks and benefits of HRT was not as controversial as it is nowadays. After all, most physicians and patients agreed that menopausal symptoms could impair a woman's ability to function well and enjoy her quality of life. Meanwhile, research studies and clinical experience with HRT demonstrated that the core complaints about menopause—particularly vasomotor symptoms but also sexual problems and overall quality of life—could be addressed with HRT. Beyond its help in relieving symptoms, HRT was also seen as an essential strategy for the prevention of problems possibly confronting a woman in her postmenopausal years: cardiovascular disease, stroke, osteoporosis, hip fractures, colon cancer, dementia, and so on. With all these potential advantages in mind, perimenopausal women and their physicians embraced HRT, sometimes without a systematic approach to what hormone formulation or preparation to use, when or why to use it, and when or how to stop it. Then came the WHI tsunami.

The Women's Health Initiative

In recent years, people have become polarized over the use of menopausal hormone therapy, primarily as a result of the findings of the Women's Health Initiative (WHI) (Rossouw et al. 2002). The goal of this federally funded research project was to examine many aspects of women's health—from nutrition to dementia—during menopause in more than 160,000 women. The most famous and controversial part of the WHI was a clinical study on the risks and benefits of HRT in preventing heart disease and other health problems (Warren 2004).

The study was conducted in a way that had never been done before: women were followed and monitored over a number of years to assess whether HRT could help them avoid the development of health problems. The clinical trial component of this initiative, which started in the late 1990s, included more than 16,000 women on a specific combination of hormones (conjugated estrogen plus progestin) that was widely used in the United States at that time. The trial also included a group of women who were given a placebo (like a sugar pill) and another group of women who received estrogen alone (these were women who'd had their uterus removed and therefore did not need progesterone to protect their endometrial lining).

The key point about the WHI trial is that it was not a treatment study for women suffering from vasomotor and other symptoms during the menopausal transition. Rather, it was a prevention study focused on helping postmenopausal women avoid heart disease (and perhaps hip fractures, osteoporosis, and dementia) with the use of HRT. As a prevention study, the safety standards were very high, which means any indication that the treatment was causing more harm than good would be red-flagged immediately. In 2002, about five years into the clinical trial, the researchers decided to stop the intervention because they had noted a slightly increased risk (calculated as the number of extra cases per 10,000 women per year) for breast cancer (eight extra cases) and cardiovascular events, such as stroke (seven extra cases), heart attacks (six extra cases), and blood clots (eighteen extra cases), in women receiving HRT compared to a placebo. There were also observable benefits, such as fewer hip fractures (minus five cases) or colon cancers (minus six cases) with HRT. Overall, most postmenopausal women felt confused, almost betrayed, by so much conflicting information over the course of years. There was a sense of panic disseminated through the media (lay and professional), and the first reaction of some patients and physicians was to stop using or prescribing HRT altogether.

Now, almost ten years after the trial was halted (a decade into the post-WHI era), the clinical trial design, its conclusions, and possible misinterpretations have been the subject of much reflection and discussion. Here's what you need to know about the WHI to better understand what we now consider a safe use of HRT, or *menopause hormone therapy* (MHT), as it is now called:

- Women in the WHI study were on average more than sixty-three years old, which means they were many years into the postmenopausal period. Most physicians agree that the results of the WHI study do not apply to all women and particularly to women who are entering menopause.

- A third of women in the WHI study were obese, a third were hypertensive, almost half were smokers, and about 15 percent were on medications for high cholesterol. We should not extrapolate data gathered from an overall unhealthy older menopausal population and apply it to younger (and hopefully healthier) women seeking treatment for menopausal symptoms.

- The WHI study did not assess the efficacy and safety of hormone treatments for menopausal symptoms (hot flashes, night sweats) in women making the transition to menopause. More recent studies have now shown the efficacy and safety of various hormone preparations or combinations (Buster 2010).

After many years of looking at the WHI results and careful review of other study findings, the consensus is that hormone therapy should still be considered a good choice for some women, but for each woman and her doctor, the question remains: for whom and for how long?

You may be already on hormone therapy, or you may be questioning whether hormone therapy could help you. For starters, pay attention to the changes you have noticed and the symptoms you recorded in your weekly menopause symptom diary. This information will guide you as you look at different treatment options.

When Hormone Therapy Makes Sense

The risks and benefits of hormone therapy will depend on your personal situation and must take into account your health status and risk factors. You will need to discuss with your doctor (primary care physician or gynecologist) whether hormone therapy is a viable option for you.

Whether hormone therapy makes sense may be largely a matter of timing. Here are a few basic principles based on the WHI and other studies of the past decade or so:

- The best use of hormone therapy is for the alleviation of menopausal symptoms (particularly hot flashes and night sweats) in younger (perimenopausal, early postmenopausal) women. Hormones are still the gold standard treatment for hot flashes (North American Menopause Society 2010a).

- The use of hormones, either systemic (by mouth or via skin) or local (intravaginal), can help alleviate urogenital or sexual complaints, such as vaginal atrophy or dryness. Quite often these symptoms are associated with pain during sexual intercourse (North American Menopause Society 2010a).

- The most beneficial, cost-effective time for hormone therapy seems to be within the first ten years of the menopause transition or before sixty years of age, whichever comes first. For example, analyses of WHI data by age or time since menopause find that an increased risk for heart disease with hormone therapy was confined to older women or those who used hormones in their late menopausal years. Younger women saw no increased risk but instead saw a trend toward benefit. The decision to stay on or initiate hormones needs to be carefully reviewed with your physician and tailored to your needs and risks (Harman et al. 2011).

- Women in their sixties and seventies may still want hormones, to alleviate their symptoms and maintain a good quality of life. Taking hormones at this age will require closer monitoring, however, and we recommend considering other options.

- Not all hormonal preparations are the same. Several estrogens and progestins are available and can be administered in different ways: orally, transdermally, and locally. They also may differ in their cost, side effects, and impact on your physical or emotional symptoms, as well as in how your body metabolizes them.

Hormone treatment may be right for you. If you are considering hormone treatment, you will want to discuss this option with your doctor and base your decision on your overall health conditions and what symptoms you want to target. For example, a form of estrogen called *estradiol* in patches or gel has been shown to be particularly helpful in alleviating mood symptoms. You should review all the available options before making your choice, and be prepared to try alternatives if necessary.

ALTERNATIVES

If you find yourself still struggling with symptoms despite the use of hormone therapy, or if you are unable or unwilling to try hormones to ease your symptoms, there are other options.

Lifestyle Changes

Certain lifestyle changes have been shown to be effective in reducing hot flashes, although with modest results (Albertazzi 2007). For example, reducing alcohol and caffeine intake, quitting smoking, changing ambient temperature (by keeping your living room or bedroom a bit cooler), and eating less spicy foods may all help. Reducing alcohol and caffeine intake or quitting smoking if you are a smoker will result in some additional benefits to your overall health and quality of life.

Antidepressants

Antidepressants are multifaceted medications that can sometimes not only improve mood symptoms but also help alleviate anxiety, pain, and hot flashes. The rationale behind the use of antidepressants for menopausal symptoms comes from the involvement of neurotransmitters, particularly serotonin and norepinephrine, in controlling your body's temperature (a process called *thermoregulation*). Your body temperature is regulated by a series of complex mechanisms that include thermal sensors in your body and the hypothalamus, located in the brain. All these mechanisms are fine-tuned to keep your temperature within a very narrow range called the *thermoneutral zone* or *homeostatic range*. When they are unbalanced, your body temperature crosses the upper or lower threshold of this homeostatic range and causes you to experience sweating or chills. It turns out that both serotonin and norepinephrine can influence thermoregulation, through either the hypothalamus or the sensors in your body.

Several antidepressants that primarily influence serotonin or serotonin and norepinephrine transmission (called serotonin-specific reuptake inhibitors [SSRIs] or serotonin-norepinephrine reuptake inhibitors

[SNRIs]) have also been studied for the treatment of hot flashes and showed good results even in nondepressed patients. There are studies showing good efficacy and tolerability with paroxetine (Paxil, Paxil CR) (Stearns et al. 2003); venlafaxine (Effexor XR) (Evans et al. 2005); sertraline (Zoloft) (Gordon et al. 2006); fluoxetine (Prozac) (Suvanto-Luukkonen et al. 2005); escitalopram (Cipralex, Lexapro) (Freeman, Guthrie, et al. 2011); and desvenlafaxine (Pristiq) (Archer et al. 2009). Other antidepressants, such as duloxetine (Cymbalta) and quetiapine (Seroquel XR), have also alleviated hot flashes in smaller studies (Hall, Frey, and Soares 2011).

If you are considering using an antidepressant to treat hot flashes, you may want to discuss the pros and cons of this option with your doctor. In some cases, antidepressants may affect your sexual satisfaction by reducing or delaying your ability to achieve an orgasm. Other side effects include excessive sedation or insomnia, drowsiness, headaches, and weight gain. On the other hand, a low dose may work well with little or no side effects. Sometimes you may even benefit from the side effects that accompany the use of a certain antidepressant. For example, if you have trouble sleeping, an antidepressant that causes drowsiness might help you get more sleep, which will also help with your other symptoms.

Antidepressants are not known to be particularly helpful for urogenital symptoms, except in some cases for urinary incontinence. But if you happen to suffer from hot flashes, and especially if you also experience depression or anxiety, antidepressants may be particularly helpful.

Other Medications

Other medications have been successfully used for the treatment of hot flashes during menopause. Gabapentin (Neurontin, Fanatrex) and clonidine (Catapres) are among those with more efficacy and safety data supporting their use. Note that these medications were not originally developed for the treatment of menopausal symptoms and may also cause side effects. Gabapentin was originally developed for the treatment of epilepsy and also used for neuropathic pain. Although generally well tolerated in doses used for hot flashes (lower than for other indications), potential side effects are headaches, dizziness, and disorientation (brain fogginess). Clonidine was originally developed for high blood pressure, with use in pain conditions and anxiety as well. Side effects include dizziness if blood pressure goes too low, as well as dry mouth, constipation, dizziness, or sleep problems. It is generally well tolerated in doses used for hot flashes (also lower than for other indications). These drugs should be used under the guidance of your doctor and require an appropriate assessment of risks and benefits and choice of an adequate prescribed dosing.

Complementary and Alternative Methods

Many women are now opting for the use of complementary and alternative methods (CAMs) due to their concerns about negative side effects, tolerability, and/or safety of hormonal or nonhormonal medical interventions. It is remarkable that CAMs have become so popular and are often sold over-the-counter though the research on their safety and effectiveness is limited. Such so-called natural options are not without risk, particularly when used in combination with other prescribed medications. Here are some of the most frequently used CAMs and evidence for each of these agents for the management of menopausal symptoms.

BLACK COHOSH

Overall, the evidence for the efficacy of black cohosh for the treatment of vasomotor symptoms is contradictory, with some positive and many negative studies; nonetheless, this compound has been widely used, particularly in some European countries. It is important to note that there are significant differences among preparations and dosages of black cohosh on the market or used across clinical studies. Importantly, a well-done study comparing black cohosh with a placebo, estrogen, or other botanicals did not reveal a significant benefit of this treatment for the management of hot flashes over the course of one year (Newton et al. 2006).

RED CLOVER

Several studies have investigated red clover as a potential treatment for vasomotor symptoms in menopausal women. Red clover is a source of *isoflavones*, one of three types of plant-derived compounds called *phytoestrogens*. These compounds have estrogen-like and anti-estrogen-like effects. Promensil, an over-the-counter preparation of red clover isoflavone extracts, was used in most studies and showed limited therapeutic effects for the reduction of hot flash severity or frequency (Knight, Howes, and Eden 1999; Tice et al. 2003).

SAINT-JOHN'S-WORT

Most studies with Saint-John's-wort included women with mild or less frequent hot flashes. These studies showed a moderate reduction in symptoms and suggested that Saint-John's-wort may be effective in the treatment of vasomotor symptoms (Abdali, Khajehei, and Tabatabaee 2010). For women complaining of mood symptoms and vasomotor symptoms, this might be a valid treatment option, as long as the benefits and potential side effects are carefully considered.

ACUPUNCTURE

A few studies have suggested that acupuncture can be used for the treatment of vasomotor symptoms, with some limited results. Most of the improvement obtained with acupuncture in these studies was not sustained over time, except in patients with other complaints, such as insomnia and chronic pain (Borud et al. 2010; Kim et al. 2010).

OMEGA-3 FATTY ACIDS

A small study on the use of omega-3 fatty acids for the treatment of depressive and vasomotor symptoms in women transitioning to menopause has shown promising results (Freeman, Hibbeln, et al. 2011). The use of omega-3 fatty acids led to a reduction in mood symptoms and in frequency of hot flashes per day. It also reduced the negative impact on quality of life associated with these symptoms. Further study is needed to support the use of this treatment before it can be more generally recommended.

Cognitive Behavioral Therapy

In the next chapter, we will discuss in more detail the rationale for using CBT for the alleviation of menopausal symptoms. Since menopause-associated symptoms are quite complex in nature, the use of CBT will require a careful mapping to identify areas or symptoms that could benefit the most from this type of intervention.

If your transition to menopause is accompanied by anxiety or mood difficulties, sleep disturbances, or hot flashes, CBT may be particularly helpful, because several techniques and practical guidelines apply to these problems. We have had some promising results with CBT in alleviating hot flashes and the degree to which these symptoms affect a woman's quality of life and overall well-being (Green et al. 2010).

CONSIDERING ALL THE OPTIONS

In chapter 2, you read about four women coping with menopausal symptoms. Here's how each of these women began to address her symptoms:

Jane tried acupuncture to alleviate her hot flashes and night sweats. Although she found it quite relaxing, she didn't notice any improvement in her symptoms. She planned to talk to her doctor about whether hormone therapy might benefit her.

Catherine was open to the idea of trying an antidepressant to help alleviate her symptoms of depression. She saw her doctor and discussed her concerns. Her doctor suggested that she give CBT a try first, given the preoccupation she had with her role in life and finding her own personal meaning. They decided she would try an antidepressant later if CBT didn't work on its own.

Gloria reviewed all of her treatment options with her doctor. They decided to implement hormone therapy given that her sleep disruption seemed to be triggered initially by her night sweats. They planned to monitor her closely and discussed the possibility of adding an antidepressant to address her symptoms of anxiety if these continued to persist.

Ellen's doctor referred her to a specialized anxiety clinic where she received CBT for her panic attacks. She attended a twelve-session group and found that her anxiety symptoms were significantly reduced. She was able to start doing all of the things she had been avoiding. Partway through treatment, she realized that she felt normal again. Although she continued to experience occasional panic attacks, she no longer felt controlled by them. Her confidence was back and she felt well prepared to cope with her menopause-related anxiety symptoms.

Now that you have learned about the different treatment options for menopausal symptoms, are there any options that you want to explore further? We recommend booking an appointment with your family doctor or gynecologist to review the menopausal symptoms that you are experiencing and to explore all the treatment options available to you. The remainder of this book will focus on cognitive behavioral therapy and show you how to use CBT to address menopausal symptoms.

SUMMING IT ALL UP

- Hormone replacement therapy, also known as menopause hormone therapy, can be used to reduce menopausal symptoms and improve your quality of life, but it is not recommended for everyone.

- The Women's Health Initiative (WHI) and other studies have shown that hormone therapy is best used to alleviate menopausal symptoms in younger women who are in the perimenopausal or early postmenopausal stages, within the first ten years of the menopause transition, or before age sixty. Hormone therapy can be used in later life but requires close monitoring by a physician and careful consideration of alternative treatment options.

- One size does not fit all when it comes to hormone therapy. You should consult with your doctor to choose the therapy most suited to your needs.

- You can apply lifestyle changes to improve your menopausal symptoms, although the effects may be modest. Lifestyle changes may include reducing alcohol and caffeine, quitting smoking, turning down the thermostat in your house, and reducing your intake of spicy food.

- Antidepressants may be an effective option for addressing numerous menopausal symptoms, including mood symptoms, anxiety, pain, and hot flashes.

- So-called natural strategies may seem promising but are not necessarily safe. More studies are needed.

- Before embarking on any of the treatment options suggested in this chapter, you should discuss your unique situation with your doctor and carefully consider the benefits and risks of all your options.

- Cognitive behavioral therapy is a psychological treatment that may be particularly helpful for addressing a range of menopausal symptoms, particularly for individuals experiencing anxiety and mood difficulties, sleep disturbances, and hot flashes.

CHAPTER 4

Taking a Cognitive Behavioral Approach

What is cognitive behavioral treatment?

How can it reduce menopausal symptoms?

How can I use it to address my unique combination of symptoms?

What are the CBT strategies I can use to change how I feel?

Chapter 3 covered the different types of treatments for menopause and the pros and cons associated with each. Perhaps you have tried some of these treatments in the past and have stopped for various reasons. Maybe you are currently using one or more of these treatments but are unsatisfied as your symptoms continue to disrupt your life. Whatever your reasons, you are interested in trying a cognitive behavioral approach, either alone or in combination with one or more other treatments. It's time to begin!

HOW CBT WORKS

Cognitive behavioral therapy has been extensively investigated in research studies and shown to be highly effective for reducing symptoms across a range of problems and health-related conditions, including depression, anxiety disorders, marital distress, anger, chronic pain, and eating disorders, such as bulimia nervosa (Butler et al. 2006). It has just recently been applied to reducing menopausal symptoms, with promising effects (Green et al. 2010).

CBT is based on the idea that your thoughts and your behaviors play an important role in determining how you feel. It is also based on the idea that by choosing how to respond to a particular situation, you have the power to control how you feel. For example, consider the symptoms of a hot flash and how two people may cope differently with this experience:

Jane found unexpected hot flashes embarrassing. She began avoiding social situations, such as dinner parties or eating in restaurants, because she was concerned that people would take notice and make comments. Although she never knew when she was going to have a hot flash, she often found herself worrying about even the possibility of it occurring. Her worry consumed a lot of her energy in the time leading up to a social event and really took away from her ability to relax and enjoy herself.

Gloria also experienced unexpected hot flashes that caused her to sweat profusely and feel uncomfortable. She often reminded herself that eventually these symptoms would pass. When people would make comments or seem to take notice, she would make a joke about having a hot flash. She also carried a small towel in her purse, so she felt prepared in the event that one did happen.

Both Jane and Gloria are affected by uncomfortable and unexpected hot flashes, a common symptom of menopause. However, you can see that the approach each of them takes to manage this symptom is quite different. Jane is focused on what other people think about her when she has the symptom, and she has begun avoiding social situations so that she doesn't have to cope with the possibility of one occurring. Jane's thoughts about her hot flashes (*People will think negatively of me, and I will be embarrassed*) and her behaviors (worrying and avoiding social situations) increase the negative impact this symptom has on her life.

Meanwhile, Gloria is focused on the idea that her hot flashes are temporary and an unpleasant symptom that can be managed. She deals with the symptoms when they happen and is not overly concerned about what others think. Gloria's thoughts (*I can manage this symptom; at least this hot flash won't last forever*) and behavior (carrying a small towel to use in the event of excessive sweating rather than avoiding social situations) allow her to feel prepared for coping with the unexpected nature of the symptom and also minimize the negative impact it has on her life.

These examples highlight the important role that thoughts and behaviors play in determining how you feel and cope with unpleasant experiences. This is the power of the CBT approach. You can exert control over how you feel and cope as you choose how to respond to an experience.

Taking a Step Back

Many of us go through life on autopilot, not really taking notice of how we respond to the world around us—it just happens to us. We are unaccustomed to taking a step back and examining our thoughts; we simply have them and they may seem automatic. We also do not generally examine our behaviors and how they connect to our thoughts and feelings. We just live our lives as best we can.

CBT presents us with an opportunity to take a step back and realize the power that we have over how we respond to challenges. In the next section of this book, you will learn how to examine your thoughts and shift your perspective. You will see how your thoughts play an important role in determining how you feel, both emotionally and physically. You will also become aware of the behavioral choices you tend to make as well as the range of possibilities available to you. By learning this approach, you will gain personal control over how you respond to unpleasant symptoms. You will have the ability to minimize the negative impact that menopausal symptoms may be having on your life. You have the power to change how you feel by choosing how you respond to your experience.

What You Put In Is What You Get Out

CBT is an approach that requires your active participation to be successful. In addition to providing a way to understand your symptoms, CBT involves learning specific strategies designed to reduce your symptoms and enhance your well-being. You will need to set aside time to learn and practice these strategies so that you can enjoy the benefits of reducing your menopausal symptoms and minimizing the negative impact they have had on your life. Unlike taking a medication, where the benefits cease when the medication is discontinued, the benefits of CBT will last long after you have finished learning how to use the strategies in this book. People often find themselves applying these strategies to many areas of their life.

A major part of CBT is increasing your awareness of your symptoms and your associated thoughts, feelings, and behaviors. With this information, you can then use CBT to target problematic thoughts and behaviors, reduce the negative impact of your symptoms and associated distress, and feel more in control of your life. Another important part is learning more about the nature of the symptoms you are experiencing, as you've been doing in this book. With a better understanding of the changes that are happening to your body, you will feel more in control. For instance, understanding the physical reasons for your hot flashes might reduce your anxiety when you experience them, as you will know what is happening to your body. In addition, this knowledge could help you prepare for these symptoms—as you apply cognitive and behavioral strategies from part 2—in turn reducing their frequency and intensity. To begin this journey, take a look at the CBT model (figure 4.1).

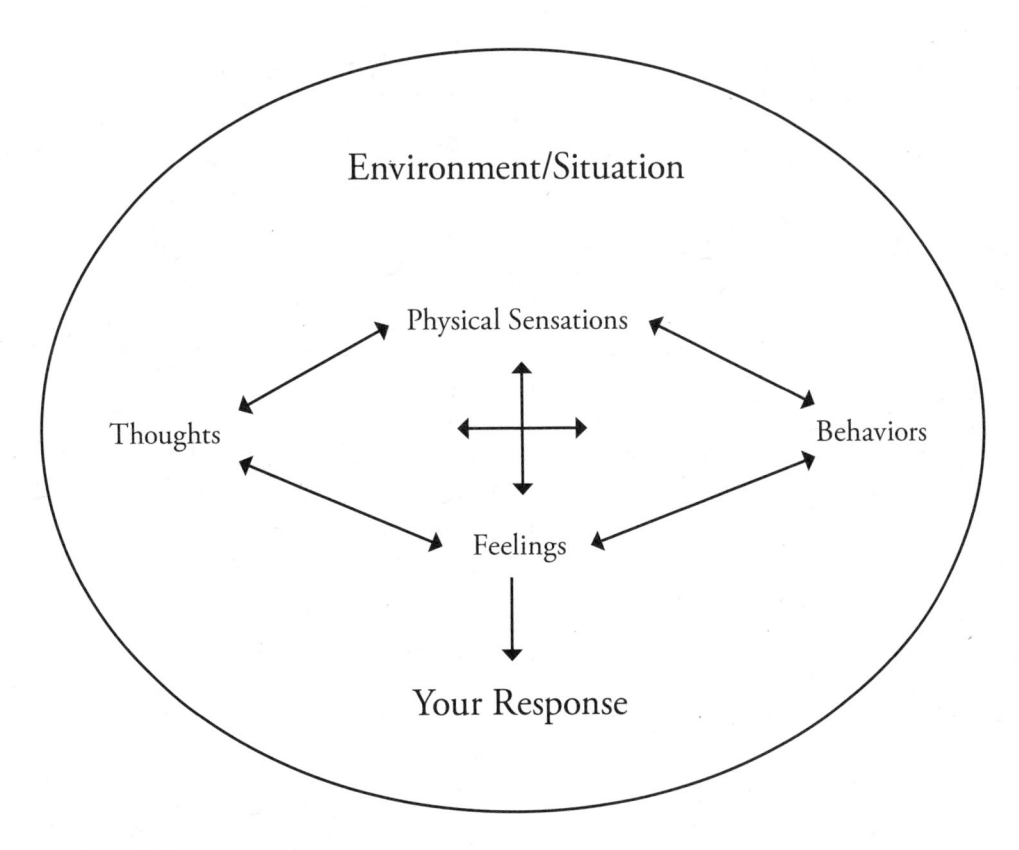

Figure 4.1: The CBT model

In this figure, you can see that your physical sensations (or symptoms), thoughts, feelings, and behaviors are represented as different components that occur within the larger environment, or context. These components are interconnected, which means that if you change one component, you can possibly affect each of the other components in the model; for example, if you change your behavior, it has the potential to change the way you think, how you feel, and the physical sensations that you experience.

The different components can interact to increase potential negative responses. They can also interact to create a more helpful or adaptive way of responding. As you begin to identify the components of your own individual response, you will be able to shift how you think, behave, and feel.

Of course, making changes requires learning new skills, and the environment you live in and situations you experience can also play a role or have an impact on you.

The examples below illustrate how these interacting connections may play out in daily life for the women who were first presented in chapter 2.

PHYSICAL SENSATIONS

Jane experienced hot flashes that were significantly disruptive. Hot flashes and other physical sensations would come under the heading of physical sensations within the CBT model. Whenever Jane experienced a hot flash, it would affect her thoughts, feelings, and behaviors.

Physical sensation ⟶ **Thoughts** (*This hot flash will last forever. This is so embarrassing. Everyone will notice.*)
(hot flashes)

Feelings (depression, stress, anxiety, and loss of control)

Behaviors (avoiding work, people, and parties)

The more Jane focused on other people's responses to her, the more her physical sensations intensified and the worse she felt. She began to avoid more and more situations. You can see how the components in the CBT model (figure 4.1) interacted with each other to increase Jane's response.

THOUGHTS

With the end of her periods, Catherine began to reflect on the choices she had made in life and started to have a number of thoughts related to this. She began to question whether she'd made the right decision to not get married or have children. These thoughts influenced her feelings, behaviors, and physical sensations.

Thoughts ⟶ **Feelings** (depressed, despairing, anxious, regretful)
(*What if I made the wrong decision?*)

Behaviors (social withdraw)

Physical sensations (loss of energy)

Taking a Cognitive Behavioral Approach

As Catherine reflected on her life and questioned her decisions, she had increasing feelings of regret and despair. In response, she became less interested in the social activities she usually engaged in. She felt exhausted physically, which made her feel even worse emotionally. Again, you can see how each of the components in the CBT model interacted to amplify Catherine's negative response.

BEHAVIORS

Ellen began to experience panic attacks when she entered late perimenopause, and she began to avoid situations where she feared she might have another attack. Although her avoidance response reduced her anxiety in the short term, because she didn't have to cope with a panic attack in the feared situation, in the long term she felt more anxious and depressed because the panic attacks were constricting her lifestyle. She started to wonder if she would ever be normal again.

Behaviors ⟶ **Feelings** (anxious, depressed)
(avoidance)

        Thoughts *(I am not normal. This anxiety will never go away. I am not in control of my life.)*

        Physical sensations (increased physical arousal, fatigue, low energy)

For Ellen, an avoidance response led to increased anxiety, increased negative thoughts, and increased physical sensations of anxiety and depression, which in turn led her to avoid social situations even more. You can see how the components represented in the CBT model interact to increase Ellen's negative response and, consequently, the impact that her symptoms were having on her life.

FEELINGS

Gloria began experiencing sleep disruption when she entered early postmenopause. Although her sleep disruption was initially caused by the physical symptom of night sweats, it was her feelings about the sleep disruption that exacerbated this symptom.

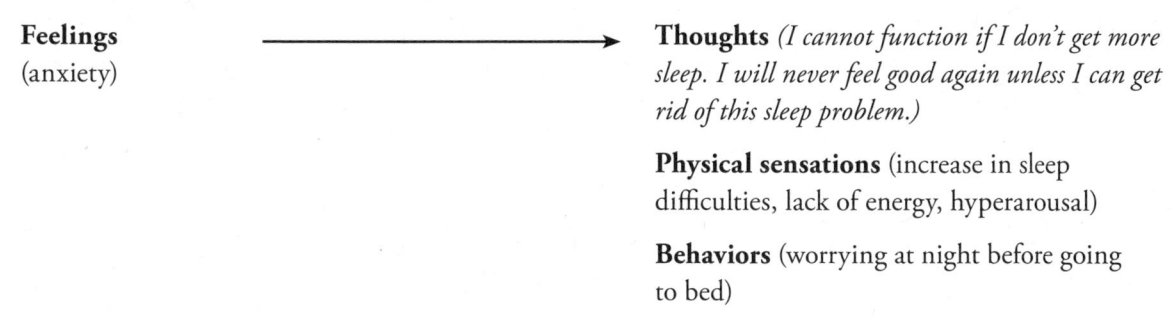

Feelings ⟶ **Thoughts** *(I cannot function if I don't get more sleep. I will never feel good again unless I can get rid of this sleep problem.)*
(anxiety)

        Physical sensations (increase in sleep difficulties, lack of energy, hyperarousal)

        Behaviors (worrying at night before going to bed)

As Gloria felt more and more pressure to get a better night's sleep, she was less likely to sleep well. Her worrying during the time that she was trying to get back to sleep increased her level of arousal and interfered with her ability to sleep. She found herself even more sleep deprived and, as a consequence, felt less physically well and less able to cope.

How to Apply the CBT Model

You can apply the CBT model to your own experience of menopausal symptoms and identify the different components of your response. The following worksheet will help you examine your menopausal symptoms over the last week. Before you complete the worksheet, you may want to make photocopies in case you want to use the worksheet in the future to gain further awareness.

CBT Model Worksheet

Reflect over the past week on the symptom(s) of menopause that you experienced, and consider them in relation to the CBT model in figure 4.1. First identify the symptom and rate your experience of this symptom in terms of severity (or intensity) on a scale of 0 to 100, where 0 is not at all severe and 100 is the most severe. Then rate the experience in terms of interference (or impact) on the same scale, where 0 is no interference and 100 is the greatest interference. Use the following rating scales as a guide:

Severity/Intensity

0   10   20   30   40   50   60   70   80   90   100

not at all severe   mildly severe   moderately severe   most severe

Interference/Impact

0   10   20   30   40   50   60   70   80   90   100

not at all interfering   mildly interfering   moderately interfering   most interfering

Next, try to recall the situation in which the symptom occurred. Then break down each experience by identifying your thoughts, feelings, behaviors, and physical sensations.

Example:

Symptom: *sleep disruption*

Severity/intensity: *70*   Interference/impact: *85*

Environment/situation: *Tuesday 3:20 a.m., awoke from a night sweat and tried to get back to sleep after I changed my nightgown.*

→ Thought(s): *If I don't sleep now, I will be so tired tomorrow. I won't be able to get things done. I will never get a good night's sleep again.*

→ Feeling(s): *anxious, irritated, frustrated, helpless*

→ Behavior(s): *worrying behavior, checking the clock to see how many hours of possible sleep are left*

→ Physical sensation(s): *fatigue, physical tension and symptoms of arousal*

Your Experience:

1. Symptom: _____

   Severity/intensity (0–100): _____   Interference/impact (0–100): _____

   Environment/situation: _____
   _____

   → Thought(s): _____
   _____

   → Feeling(s): _____
   _____

   → Behavior(s): _____
   _____

   → Physical sensation(s): _____
   _____

2. Symptom: _____

   Severity/intensity (0–100): _____   Interference/impact (0–100): _____

   Environment/situation: _____
   _____

   → Thought(s): _____
   _____

   → Feeling(s): _____
   _____

   → Behavior(s): _____
   _____

   → Physical sensation(s): _____
   _____

3. Symptom:

Severity/intensity (0–100): _____   Interference/impact (0–100): _____

Environment/situation: _____

_____

→ Thought(s): _____

_____

→ Feeling(s): _____

_____

→ Behavior(s): _____

_____

→ Physical sensation(s): _____

_____

4. Symptom:

Severity/intensity (0–100): _____   Interference/impact (0–100): _____

Environment/situation: _____

_____

→ Thought(s): _____

_____

→ Feeling(s): _____

_____

→ Behavior(s): _____

_____

→ Physical sensation(s): _____

_____

How to Use CBT

Now that you have an understanding of the CBT model and how it applies to your menopausal symptoms and experience, you can learn how to use CBT to help reduce your menopausal symptoms and the associated distress and negative impact they may be having on your life.

Figure 4.2 represents another way of understanding the CBT model and where you might intervene with troubling symptoms. Say you are out at a close friend's birthday party. You are listening to other partygoers talk about their summer vacation, and you suddenly notice that you are starting to become very hot. This is not an unfamiliar physical feeling to you. You know all too well that this is the start of another hot flash. You begin to think that others will notice your discomfort, and you feel your heart rate increase in response. As your anxiety heightens, the intensity of your hot flash increases as well. You have the thought that this experience will last forever, which further increases your anxiety. You find it increasingly difficult to concentrate on the conversation. You abruptly decide to leave the party.

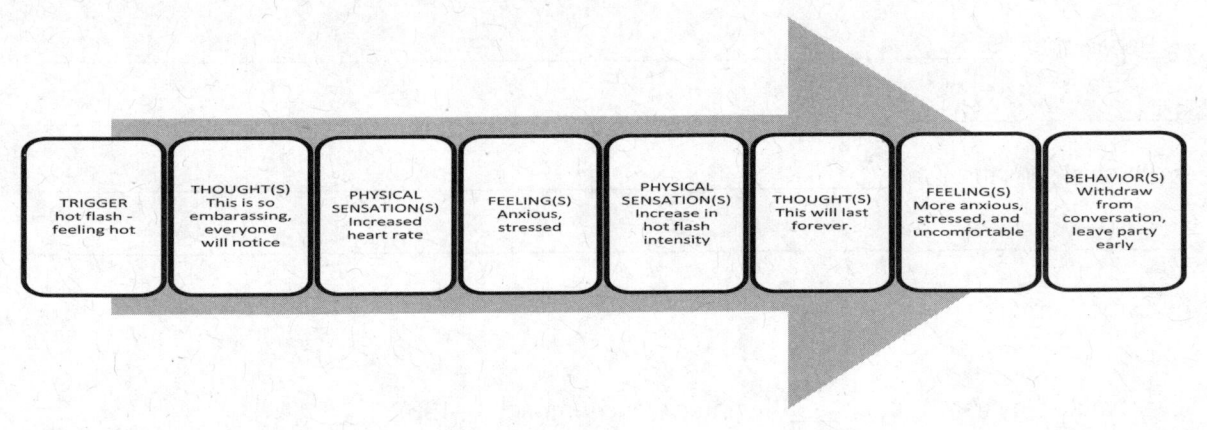

TRIGGER: hot flash - feeling hot → THOUGHT(S): This is so embarassing, everyone will notice → PHYSICAL SENSATION(S): Increased heart rate → FEELING(S): Anxious, stressed → PHYSICAL SENSATION(S): Increase in hot flash intensity → THOUGHT(S): This will last forever. → FEELING(S): More anxious, stressed, and uncomfortable → BEHAVIOR(S): Withdraw from conversation, leave party early

Figure 4.2: How CBT components interact

By using the CBT model as illustrated in figure 4.2, you can see the different connections that exist, produce symptoms, or exacerbate existing ones. So how might you intervene to reduce the impact of this troubling symptom?

Although you may want to, it's not always possible to try to eliminate the trigger, which is in this case the arrival of a hot flash. Hot flashes are a very common menopausal symptom that women experience as a result of physiological changes, and hence, they are going to occur at times. Therefore, the goal of the intervention would not be to eliminate the hot flash but rather to reduce the intensity of the symptom as well as the distress and interference that it produces. By defining this goal, you will see that, in the case of hot flashes, you could intervene at the point where you begin to have negative thoughts about your experience, which influences your behavior. Breaking down your experience in this way allows you to examine the connections between components, determine your goal, and then decide where you will implement various learned strategies and techniques to accomplish your goal.

Setting Goals

It is very important to have clearly defined goals before trying out a new treatment. Having a goal clarifies what you want to achieve and allows you to determine when you have been successful in applying the CBT approach. It is important to set realistic and attainable goals for treatment. Take, for example, someone who wants to treat his or her chronic pain. CBT has been shown to be a very effective treatment strategy for this condition. However, someone who starts CBT for chronic pain and has the goal of eliminating her pain completely will be disappointed, as this goal is unrealistic. A more realistic goal would be to reduce the severity of pain, the number of flare-ups, and the distress and interference associated with the pain.

The same is true for many of the physical symptoms of menopause, which are hormonally driven. Although it would be great if you could eliminate these symptoms altogether, this is not a realistic possibility. A more realistic goal would be to reduce the severity of your menopausal symptoms and the negative impact they may be having in your life in terms of interference and distress. So going back to the hot flash example illustrated in figure 4.2, you can use the CBT approach to change your thought from *This unpleasant hot flash will last forever*, which has a negative impact on your mood (you feel anxious, uncomfortable, and stressed) to *I can cope with this hot flash and it will soon pass*, which has less of a negative impact on your mood and allows you to continue to participate in the social event while coping with the uncomfortable menopausal symptom.

By using this approach, you can change how you feel by changing how you think and behave in response to situational triggers. To do this, you will learn a set of basic CBT strategies.

CBT STRATEGIES: THE BASICS

CBT strategies are the tools you can use to target the components of the CBT model described in the chapter. These strategies will be used in different combinations in each of the chapters in part 2, where you will learn how to apply them to address your specific goals.

Cognitive Strategies

Cognitive strategies aim to shift your perspective or way of thinking about a situation to be more realistic. In day-to-day life, you probably don't spend too much time thinking about how or what you are thinking. Most people are more focused on simply living and doing and may not even be aware of specific thoughts that play an important role in their emotional experience. By becoming more aware of your thoughts, you can take control of how you feel and respond. This is the basic premise of cognitive strategies pioneered by Aaron Beck (Beck et al. 1979) and Albert Ellis (Ellis and Harper 1961).

Once you become aware of your thoughts, you can examine them to see whether they are realistic for a given situation. We all have our own unique way of perceiving the world, influenced by our past experiences and our personality. Certain *cognitive distortions* or styles of thinking can increase the likelihood of experiencing negative emotions, such as feelings of unhappiness, depression, and anxiety. Some common types of cognitive distortions, also called *thinking errors*, have been identified (Barlow and Craske 1994; Burns 1980). The following table lists some of these cognitive distortions along with some examples.

Cognitive Distortion	Definition	Example
all-or-nothing thinking	You have a tendency to see things in extremes—as good or bad, black or white. It is a challenge for you to see the shades of gray. You may have certain standards that you believe you cannot compromise.	*I will never feel good again unless I can get rid of this sleep problem.* (Gloria)
emotional reasoning	You believe something is true because you feel it is, rather than examine the evidence to determine whether it is in fact true.	*If I think I am going to faint, I actually will.* (Ellen)
labeling/personalizing	You have a tendency to negatively judge yourself or others.	*I have been a failure in my life.* (Catherine)
jumping to conclusions/ mind reading	You have a tendency to make negative assumptions about what other people are thinking. You assume people are negatively judging you.	*If I have a hot flash, people will think negatively of me.* (Jane)
should-statements	You have a tendency to criticize yourself or others with high expectations of what you think you or others *should* or *must* do.	*I should have done more with my life.* (Catherine)
probability overestimation	You tend to predict that negative events are much more likely to happen than they realistically are.	*I will never get a good night's sleep again.* (Gloria)
catastrophizing	You believe that if a negative event occurs, the outcome will be much worse than it actually would be. You underestimate your coping abilities.	*If I have a hot flash at a meeting, that would be the worst thing ever.* (Jane)
fortune telling	You make predictions that things will turn out badly.	*Tonight will be another sleepless night.* (Gloria)
filtering	You pick out and focus on a single negative detail, dwelling on it.	*I will never experience grandchildren like my coworkers.* (Catherine)

Once you have identified a cognitive distortion, you can consider ways of viewing the situation that are more realistic and helpful. In the example described earlier in this chapter, Jane's thought that *this hot flash will last forever* illustrates the cognitive distortion of probability overestimation. Though it may feel like forever to Jane, in reality, the hot flash will last several minutes. This thought also represents the cognitive distortion of catastrophizing because Jane feels that having a hot flash would be terrible, and she has a tendency to underestimate her coping abilities. As Jane becomes aware of her tendency to overestimate negative events, catastrophize the consequences, and underestimate her coping abilities, she can start to intervene with more helpful ways of thinking.

In the chapters that follow, you will become skilled at shifting your thoughts using the following three-step approach when you experience negative emotions or symptoms in a particular situation:

1. Step back and examine your thoughts.

2. Identify an unhelpful thought or cognitive distortion.

3. Consider ways of interpreting or thinking about the situation that are more realistic.

Cognitive strategies are an important part of any CBT treatment plan, and they are even more powerful when combined with behavioral strategies.

Behavioral Strategies

Behavioral strategies aim to change what you do in response to a situation. The possibilities for new behaviors you can try are endless, and it is really a search to find the strategies that work best for you. We will provide you with many new behaviors to try with strategies geared to improve your particular symptoms.

Behavioral change requires effort because old habits are hard to break. However, the key to better coping is to keep an open mind and to actually change your behaviors by putting the strategies into practice. You will find that changing your behaviors in a strategic way will change how you think as well as how you feel.

This brings us to the next step in the process: how to personalize the approach of this book to suit your needs.

DEVELOPING A TREATMENT PLAN

The goal of this book is to offer you a treatment program for the symptoms you are experiencing right now. As you begin part 2, you will want to focus on the chapters that address your most distressing symptoms. In the next exercise, therefore, you'll develop a CBT treatment plan to outline which chapters you'll work on and in what order, as well as your treatment goals. The CBT model worksheet in this chapter, along with the symptom rating form in chapter 2, should give you all the information you need to choose which chapters in part 2 to focus on first.

The following example shows how Jane developed a CBT treatment plan to address her most distressing symptoms.

Jane's CBT Treatment Plan

Jane had rated hot flashes and mood changes as two of her most distressing symptoms. She thought about it and decided that reducing the distress and impact of hot flashes would bring about the most positive results for her, so she would begin with chapter 5, which addresses hot flashes. She also decided to work on chapters 7 and 6 to address her mood changes and anxiety, in this order:

1. Hot flashes: chapter 5

2. Mood changes: chapter 7

3. Anxiety (worries): chapter 6

She then listed her goals for each symptom. She concentrated on being realistic and making her goals achievable. She tried to answer the following questions: How would your life be different if this symptom were reduced? What would you be doing differently in your life?

Jane's goals for symptom 1:

I would like to change how I react to hot flashes. I would like to feel better able to cope when they occur instead of feeling like they are controlling my life. If I could adjust my response, I feel that I would be able to enjoy myself more and be more involved in the things I like to do instead of worrying about when the next hot flash will come and whether people will notice.

Jane's goals for symptom 2:

I would like to be happier and more involved in my life. If I weren't feeling so negative and bitter, I would be able to enjoy being with my friends and family more. I would be making plans instead of trying to find a way to get out of things.

Jane's goals for symptom 3:

I would like to stop being overly concerned about what other people think about me when I am in social settings. If I weren't worrying so much, I would have a lot more energy left to enjoy myself. I would like to concentrate on living in the moment and increase my ability to manage stresses in my life like this menopause experience.

Your CBT Treatment Plan

List your three most distressing menopausal symptoms and record the corresponding chapter that you will read to target the symptom.

1. _____: chapter _____

2. _____: chapter _____

3. _____: chapter _____

List your goals for each symptom. Remember that your goals should be specific, realistic, and achievable. Answer the following questions: How would your life be different if this symptom were reduced? What would you be doing differently in your life? How do you want to be living your life?

Goals for symptom 1:

_____

_____

_____

_____

Goals for symptom 2:

_____

_____

_____

_____

Goals for symptom 3:

_____

_____

_____

_____

Congratulations! You now have a CBT treatment plan. Now you can proceed to part 2, where you will target each of your symptoms according to your plan. Your first step will be to address the menopausal symptom that is most problematic for you in terms of severity, frequency, associated distress, or interference in your life. You are now ready to start tackling your symptoms.

SUMMING IT ALL UP

- CBT is an evidence-based psychological treatment based on the idea that you can change how you feel by changing how you think and behave in response to a given situation.

- CBT provides a framework or model for understanding your symptoms as it breaks them down into components: your physical symptoms, your thoughts, your feelings, and your behaviors. These components interact to create your response to a situation.

- CBT also involves a set of skills that you can use to target each component of your response to a given situation. It takes effort to develop these skills, but once you learn them, you can use these strategies to address the menopausal symptoms that distress you and thereby greatly improve your life.

PART 2

Cognitive Behavioral Treatment for Menopausal Symptoms

CHAPTER 5

Managing Hot Flashes and Night Sweats

What are hot flashes and night sweats?

What can I learn from monitoring my hot flashes?

What is paced respiration, and how can it help?

What other behavioral strategies can I use to reduce my hot flashes or night sweats?

What cognitive strategies can I use?

You have arrived at this chapter because you are experiencing hot flashes or night sweats and want a hand coping with these symptoms and reducing their impact on your life. Again, you need to understand the nature of any problem before you can treat it effectively. In this chapter, you'll receive some background information on the nature of vasomotor symptoms, followed by some exercises to collect some details about your personal experience of hot flashes or night sweats. Then you will learn some new cognitive and behavioral strategies for managing them.

THE FACTS ABOUT VASOMOTOR SYMPTOMS

The terms *vasomotor symptoms*, *hot flashes* (or flushes), and *night sweats* all describe the same physiological experience. The only difference between a hot flash, for instance, and a night sweat is the time when these two symptoms occur. Both are spontaneous episodes of warmth or sweating that you usually feel on your chest, neck, and face. Most of the discomfort you might feel with hot flashes comes from the intense heat dissipation when the blood vessels that are close to your skin suddenly dilate and open. You may also experience an increase in heart rate, sweating, and anxiety.

A hot flash usually lasts from one to five minutes, with a small percentage of women reporting symptoms that persist up to fifteen minutes (Kronenberg 1990). Skin temperatures return to normal gradually, usually within thirty minutes.

Prevalence

Hot flashes are the second most frequently reported perimenopausal symptom (after irregular periods), and, therefore, this symptom is considered one of the hallmarks of perimenopause (Freeman and Sherif 2007). At some time during the menopausal transition, as many as 80 percent of women will experience hot flashes and night sweats (National Institutes of Health 2005). Hot flashes can occur weekly or monthly, or even on an hourly basis, but individually, the pattern tends to be consistent.

The prevalence of this symptom differs among racial and ethnic groups. For instance, in a study that included a multiracial, multiethnic sample of women aged forty to fifty-five in the United States, African-American women reported vasomotor symptoms most frequently (45.6 percent), followed by Hispanic women (35.4 percent), Caucasian women (31.2 percent), Chinese women (20.5 percent), and Japanese women (17.6 percent) (Gold, Sternfeld, and Kelsey 2000). Some evidence suggests that body mass index (BMI) is a more important predictor of hot flashes than ethnicity, with a higher prevalence in overweight or obese women (Randolph et al. 2003).

Causes

The main theory as to why women experience hot flashes points to changes in brain chemistry, as well as a dysregulation of core body temperature, resulting from faulty temperature readings taken by sensors throughout the body and a dysregulation in the thermoregulatory system in the brain (Freedman and Roehrs 2004). This complex and delicate system involves particular areas of the brain, such as the hypothalamus, which is responsible for temperature regulation. Fluctuations in levels of estrogen, as well as changes in levels of the neurotransmitters serotonin and norepinephrine, may contribute to the emergence of hot flashes and night sweats.

Given the sensitive nature of the thermoregulatory system, increases in body temperature from physical activity or from wearing too many clothes can potentially set off a hot flash or make a hot flash more intense.

Longevity

Some women report experiencing vasomotor symptoms for anywhere between six months and two years, although other reports suggest that symptoms persist on average for three to five years (Kronenberg 1990). It's uncommon for women to experience hot flashes for more than ten years after menopause (Col et al. 2009).

SELF-MONITORING

Now that you have a good understanding of what a hot flash is, it's time to look at your personal experience of this symptom. To get a better picture, you can keep a diary for a couple of weeks to capture as many situations or circumstances during which a hot flash occurs. The information you collect will reflect the relationships within the CBT model, seen again in figure 5.1.

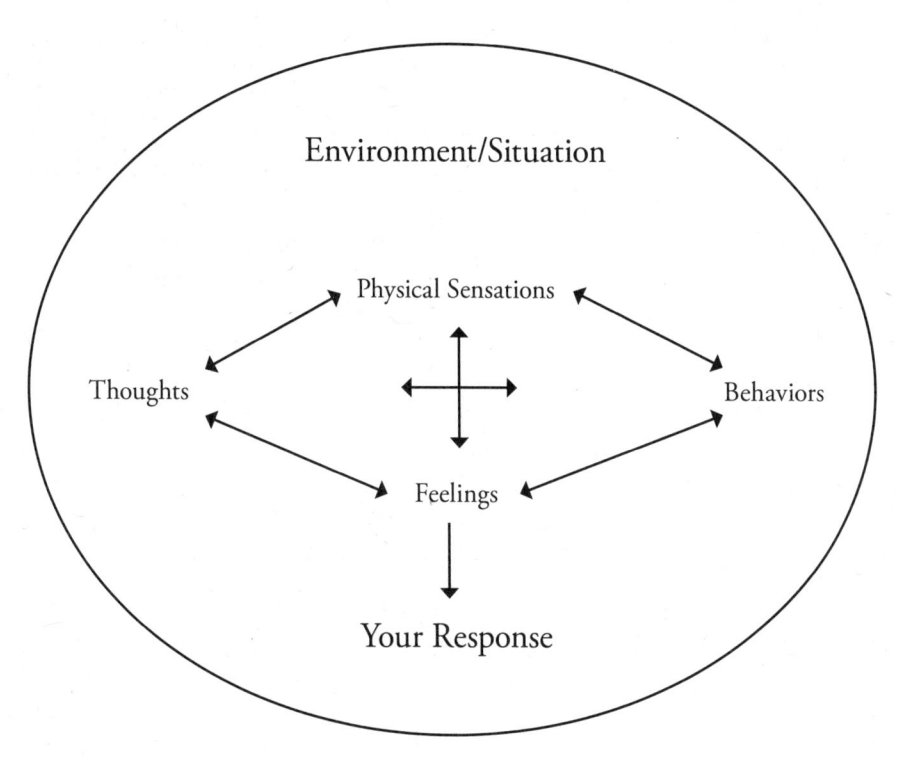

Figure 5.1: The CBT model

The Cognitive Behavioral Workbook for Menopause

The following entries from Jane's hot flash diary show how she recorded her experience with hot flashes.

Jane's Hot Flash Diary

Situation	Intensity (0–100)	Distress (0–100)	Emotions and Physical Sensations	Thoughts	Behaviors
Saturday: Shopping at the mall in the afternoon with my daughter	60	70	Frustration, uncomfortable, hot, sweaty, shaky, lightheaded	This will never end! Something is wrong with me. This is ruining my day with my daughter.	Left the store I was in right away. Took off my coat. Walked outside to cool off.
Wednesday: Contributing to an afternoon meeting with colleagues at work	50	90	Incompetent, embarrassment, hot, sweaty, lightheaded, shaky	Everyone can tell that I'm having a hot flash. I should find an excuse to miss the next meeting.	Stopped speaking and contributing as much as I usually do. Pulled my sweater closed, so no one could see me sweat.

You can use the following template to create your own hot flash diary. Before you get started, you may want to make several photocopies, so you can record all of your experiences over a two-week period.

Your Hot Flash Diary

Over the next two weeks, monitor your hot flash symptoms in the following format. List the situation (day of the week, time of day, what you were doing, whom you were with, and where you were). Rate how intense the hot flash was on a scale of 0 to 100, where 0 is not at all intense and 100 is the most intense. Also rate how much distress the hot flash caused you on a scale of 0 to 100, where 0 is the least distress and 100 is the most distress. (Note that intensity and distress levels can be independent of each other; for example, you might have a really intense hot flash but not be too distressed if no one were around to see you sweating or fanning yourself.) Also record your emotions and physical sensations, your thoughts (what was going through your mind before and after), and the behaviors that you engaged in (your response).

Situation	Intensity (0–100)	Distress (0–100)	Emotions and Physical Sensations	Thoughts	Behaviors

Analyzing the Data

After you've detailed your experiences of hot flashes for two weeks, you can analyze the data to guide your strategies for managing this symptom. This will require examining each entry in your diary and looking for any cognitive and behavioral patterns. Here's what Jane learned from this exercise.

Jane's Analysis of Her Hot Flash Diary

1. Were certain situations more distressing for you than others? If yes, which ones, and why were they more distressing?

   Yes, definitely! When I experienced a hot flash when I was around colleagues, whether at work or socializing, I became more distressed than when I had one by myself, with my immediate family, or even near strangers.

2. Were your hot flashes more intense in certain situations than in others? If yes, when were they more intense and why?

   Looking at my hot flash diary, it seems as though my hot flashes were more intense when I was involved in a physical activity, even walking in a mall with my daughter. It really was hot in there with the large crowd during the Christmas season, and I was wearing my winter coat indoors, so I wouldn't have to carry it.

3. What typical behaviors did you engage in when the hot flash occurred? Did these responses work for you? Were they disruptive or interfering? Were they supportive? Would you like to change any of your behavioral responses? Which ones?

   When I experienced a hot flash, I tended to withdraw from whatever I was doing. When I was around colleagues, I ended up withdrawing socially and not contributing that much to the conversation. I really felt like finding a way to escape the situation entirely. I think this kind of behavior can be very disruptive as it minimizes the input I give during important meetings (if I am there at all). If I experience a hot flash around my family, it can also be disruptive as it interferes with whatever I'm engaged in and I get very frustrated with that. I would like to be able to handle these situations better with new coping strategies that are not so interfering. I would like to be able to get less worked up.

4. In reviewing your diary, do you see a connection between your thoughts, your behaviors, and your feelings? How do these components interrelate when you experience a hot flash? How do you think these things affect one another when you experience a hot flash?

Definitely! Depending on the situation in which the hot flash occurs, I can feel very self-conscious, such as at work, which leads to feelings of incompetence. But if I am involved in an activity with family or around the house, I tend to get very frustrated. I noticed that the physical symptoms come first, and then I focus on them and notice more physical symptoms. I start to question myself and get in my head as I turn my attention away from what I am doing and more toward how I am feeling. This makes me feel disconnected from what I am doing and ineffective or frustrated.

5. Do you see any patterns in your experience?

I can see how different situations impact how I feel (frustrated versus incompetent), how I think ("others will notice," as opposed to "this is ruining my day"), and what I do (focus on trying to avoid instead of trying to cool down).

Your Analysis of Your Hot Flash Diary

Review the entries in your diary and answer the following questions:

1. Were certain situations more distressing for you than others? If yes, which ones, and why were they more distressing?

   _____
   _____
   _____
   _____
   _____
   _____
   _____

2. Were your hot flashes more intense in certain situations than in others? If yes, when were they more intense and why?

   _____
   _____
   _____
   _____
   _____
   _____
   _____

3. What typical behaviors did you engage in when the hot flash occurred? Did these responses work for you? Were they disruptive or interfering? Were they supportive? Would you like to change any of your behavioral responses? Which ones?

   _____
   _____

4. In reviewing your diary, do you see a connection between your thoughts, your behaviors, and your feelings? How do these components interrelate when you experience a hot flash? How do you think these things affect one another when you experience a hot flash?

5. Do you see any patterns in your experience?

BEHAVIORAL STRATEGIES FOR COPING WITH HOT FLASHES

By now, you should have a better understanding of your whole hot flash experience, including patterns of thoughts, feelings, and behaviors. For example, you may have recognized the strength of connections between certain situations in which you experience a hot flash and how you think, or how the thoughts that you experience during a hot flash can have a significant influence on how you are feeling at the moment.

It's worth paying some attention to the connection between the hot flash you experience and the behavior that you engage in. That is, what do you typically do when a hot flash occurs? Do you escape a situation or avoid one altogether? Do you start removing layers and take a drink of water? In the previous exercise, you were asked to review the typical behaviors you engage in when a hot flash occurs and if you would like to change how you respond.

You can try some different behavioral strategies to replace old ones that you've determined are ineffective. The idea behind this approach is quite simple: if you change one component in your experience of a hot flash, it has the potential to change the other components as well. For example, if Jane had decided not to wear her heavy winter coat while walking in the mall, she may not have had the hot flash in the first place, or her hot flash may have been less severe.

Changing your behavioral response to uncomfortable hot flash symptoms has the power to change how you think and feel. Furthermore, since it is not always possible to leave or avoid situations when a hot flash occurs, it's helpful to use coping strategies that can increase your tolerance of the experience while it is happening. Paced respiration is a simple behavioral technique that has been shown to substantially reduce the negative impact of a hot flash (Freedman et al. 1995).

Paced Respiration

Paced respiration is a slow, controlled diaphragmatic breathing technique. The goal is to replace chest breathing (quick and shallow) with slow, deep, abdominal breathing. This type of breathing has been used to help reduce anxiety or tension and is also a technique shown to help women control and even reduce the incidence of hot flashes (Freedman et al. 1995; Freedman and Woodward 1992). With deep abdominal breathing, your diaphragm moves downward and causes your belly to rise. With shallow breathing, your chest and shoulders will rise.

Quick Check

Place one hand on your chest, the other on your belly, and pay attention to which hand rises as you breathe normally. If the hand on your chest rises more, you are engaged more in chest breathing. If the hand on your belly rises more, you are engaged in diaphragmatic breathing.

The next exercise will help you learn to breathe from your diaphragm, using paced respiration (see figure 5.2), to reduce the distress as well as the duration of a hot flash when you have one.

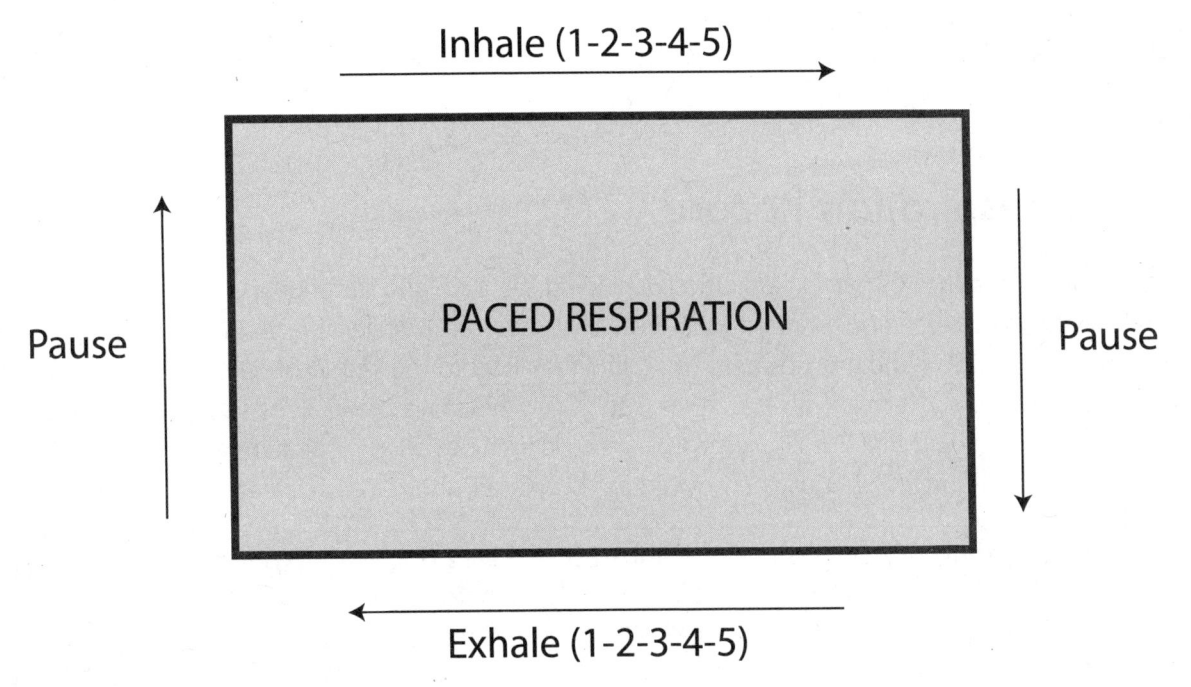

```
         Inhale (1-2-3-4-5)
        ──────────────────▶
   ▲                              │
   │                              │
Pause      PACED RESPIRATION     Pause
   │                              │
   │                              ▼
        ◀──────────────────
         Exhale (1-2-3-4-5)
```

Figure 5.2: Paced respiration

How to Use Paced Respiration

Do the following:

1. Inhale slowly through your nose to the count of five.

2. Pause for a moment.

3. Exhale slowly to the count of five.

4. Pause for a moment.

5. Repeat for ten cycles (or until your symptoms have passed).

   Keep your breathing smooth and regular.
   Practice this exercise multiple times throughout the day. Practice initially at times when you are already feeling calm and relaxed. After you become comfortable with this technique, practice it when you sense the early signs of a hot flash and continue until the sensation has passed.

You can use the following space to track your experience of paced respiration whenever you use it and especially at the first signs of a hot flash. Tracking your experience will help you determine whether this behavioral strategy is a helpful and effective one for you.

Paced Respiration Record

Record your experience of paced respiration, including the date and situation in which you practice it. Before using this technique, record your level of distress on a scale of 0 to 100, where 0 is the least distress and 100 is the most distress you could feel. Record the length of time you practice and your level of distress afterward on a scale of 0 to 100, where 0 is the least distress and 100 is the most distress you could feel. Finally, record your experience of paced respiration after practicing it, including any thoughts or feelings you noticed as you were using paced respiration.

Date and Situation	Distress Before (0–100)	Length of Time Practiced	Distress After (0–100)	Experience

After you track your experience several times, you can determine if this technique has been helpful or effective. If your level of distress was typically lower after practicing paced respiration, you may want to consider permanently adding this tool to your toolbox of strategies for coping with hot flashes.

Experimenting with Behavioral Strategies

Several behavioral strategies have been shown to be helpful in addressing hot flash symptoms, and it's worth experimenting with them to see what works for you. You may want to consider the various situations in which you experience hot flashes and which of these strategies might be worth trying. At the end of the following list of suggestions is a blank space where you can write down any other strategy that comes to mind.

Layering your clothing: Dress in layers or bring along items of clothing to easily put on and take off as needed (Kronenberg and Barnard 1992). For instance, whenever Catherine went to work, she made sure that she dressed in layers as she found that the classrooms, the staff room, and school offices were different temperatures. When too warm, she would take off a layer and was more comfortable. This made her hot flashes more tolerable, and she felt she was more in control of this symptom.

Adjusting the room temperature: You can adjust the temperature of your environment to make it more comfortable for you. You can turn off the heat or turn on air conditioning, open a window or door, or turn on a fan. This strategy may be less feasible if you live with other people and will work better in environments that you control, such as your bedroom or office (Kronenberg and Barnard 1992). Gloria found this strategy helpful, at least during the day when most of the other family members were at work or school. When they left in the morning, she either opened some windows or adjusted the thermostat to the temperature that suited her best. Gloria also got creative at night, asking her husband to sleep with another blanket so that she could open the window while sharing the same bed.

Modifying your diet: Certain foods can affect your core body temperature, such as spicy foods, hot and cold beverages, and substances containing caffeine. Consider adjusting your consumption of these types of foods to increase your comfort (Kronenberg and Barnard 1992). Although Ellen was a big fan of ethnic foods, she found that whenever she indulged, her hot flashes increased in frequency and severity. Strategically, she decided to limit her intake to once or twice a week or during times when she felt that having a hot flash would be more tolerable.

Using cold devices: Items from your freezer, such as frozen packs, ice cubes, cold cloths, and frozen bottled water, can be used in a strategic way within a given situation. Jane found it helpful to put a frozen bottle of water in her purse in the morning as she went to work. She took it into meetings with her and found that although the ice had partially melted, the coolness of the bottle on her hand helped offset any hot flash that she might experience. By reducing her hot flash symptoms, Jane found she was less self-conscious and had more confidence. She was able to focus more on meetings and less on her bodily symptoms (Freedman 2005).

Adjusting your bedroom environment: Make changes that can keep you more comfortable in the case of a night sweat. Consider the material your pajamas are made of and the bedding you are using. Are there cooler materials you could use? Adjust the thermostat if possible. Consider using a fan or opening and closing doors and windows to modulate the room temperature (Eichling 2002). Besides opening the window at night, Gloria found wearing loose cotton pajamas coupled with a single sheet for a bedcover to be the perfect combination. She kept an extra layer next to her bed in the event that she felt a bit chilled during the night.

Adjusting your activity level: Recognize the times when you are more active, and adjust your activity level to prevent a surge in body temperature. For instance, allow yourself more time in the morning to get out the door if you are usually rushed, which can increase your body temperature. Ellen was always in a hurry trying to get ready for work in the morning. She found that by getting up fifteen minutes earlier, she was able to slow down a bit and still catch the subway at the same time.

Paced respiration: Engage in this strategy any time you notice a hot flash coming on or any other time you want to calm or relax yourself (Freedman and Woodward 1992). Jane found this strategy particularly helpful when she was in the middle of a meeting and could not just get up and leave with the onset of another hot flash. After removing layers and engaging in paced respiration, she found the experience a little more tolerable and she could continue to contribute to the meeting.

Other: _____

_____

The following exercise will allow you to experiment with these different strategies. You won't know if a particular strategy will be helpful or not until you have used it, so you may want to try them all. It's also a good idea to try any strategy several times before making a final decision about it. As you modify your behavior and keep track of the results, you will see the direct impact a chosen strategy has on your symptoms.

Behavioral Modification Experiment

Choose a behavioral strategy from the list provided in this chapter (or one that you've thought of that wasn't on the list). Write down the date that you will apply the new strategy, as well as the behavior or technique you've chosen to use. After modifying your behavior, write down the outcome (Did you notice any change and, if so, was this strategy helpful?). When you are ready to move on, choose another strategy to experiment with, record the results, and continue this exercise until you've tried out all the strategies that you think might work for you.

Date	Behavior/Technique Chosen	Outcome: Helpful or Not

After this experiment, you should know which new strategies are helpful. You can adapt your behavior accordingly to reduce the frequency of hot flashes or their impact on your life.

COGNITIVE STRATEGIES FOR COPING WITH HOT FLASHES

The thoughts you have during a hot flash may increase its negative impact. For example, you may recall some of the thoughts that Jane recorded in her hot flash diary, such as *This will never end!* and *Everyone can tell that I'm having a hot flash.* These thoughts were distorted from reality and so were probably making the impact of Jane's hot flashes worse than if she weren't having these thoughts.

Countering Your Distressing Thoughts

Like Jane, you may have thoughts that make your hot flashes seem worse, but you can counter your distressing thoughts. The first step is to become aware of the thoughts you're having and identify if they are distorted. If they are, the next step is to label them, using the list of cognitive distortions from chapter 4: all-or-nothing thinking, emotional reasoning, labeling/personalization, jumping to conclusions/mind reading, should-statements, probability overestimation, catastrophizing, filtering, and fortune telling. For example, each of Jane's thoughts can be categorized as both catastrophizing and probability overestimation. The final step is to come up with alternative ways of thinking.

QUESTIONS TO CHALLENGE YOUR THINKING

Here are some questions you can use to challenge your thinking whenever a hot flash occurs:

- "Based on my own experience, what is the realistic likelihood of this negative event happening?"
- "If this negative event did happen, how bad would it really be?"
- "What strengths and coping abilities do I have to help me manage this challenging situation?"
- "What advice would a close family member or friend give to me for dealing with this situation?"
- "How would my close family member or friend handle this situation?"
- "What is the worst thing that could happen in this situation? How bad would it really be?"
- "Is this thought a realistic concern that I need to find a solution for?"
- "Is this a helpful way of looking at the situation? Is there another way of seeing things that would be more helpful?"
- "Is this my distress talking? If I were not distressed, how would I think differently about this situation?"

Asking yourself these questions can help you come up with some alternative ways of thinking.

KEEPING A THOUGHT RECORD

Keeping a thought record can help you assess your thoughts, find cognitive distortions, and come up with alternative thoughts when appropriate. The following thought record shows how Jane did this exercise with some of her thoughts about hot flashes.

Jane's Thought Record

Situation	Feelings (0–100)	Thoughts/ Predictions	Cognitive Distortions	Alternative Thoughts
Wednesday: Contributing to an afternoon meeting with colleagues at work	incompetent (80)	Everyone can tell I'm having a hot flash. I should find an excuse to miss the next meeting as this will always happen.	mind reading should-statement fortune-telling	Even though someone asked me if I was okay, they were genuinely concerned, not appalled, and seemed motivated to help ease my discomfort if I asked. Others may notice my hot flash, but it is not as bad as it seems or I believe it to be and they are likely compassionate in their response. Although people were looking at me when I spoke or took off my coat, it doesn't mean they all noticed my sweating.

You can use the following thought record to help reduce your distress during hot flashes. You may want to make several photocopies in advance, so you can use this worksheet whenever you have a hot flash that is distressing for you. With practice, you may find yourself recognizing cognitive distortions and coming up with alternative thoughts automatically as you feel a hot flash coming on.

Your Thought Record

Record each situation when you experience a distressing hot flash. Write down your feelings and rate them on a scale of 0 to 100 (where 0 is the least intense and 100 is the most intense). Record your thoughts and predictions. Then label your cognitive distortions and come up with some alternative, more realistic ways of thinking that will make you feel better. To help counter your thinking, you may want to use the list of questions provided earlier.

Situation	Feelings (0–100)	Thoughts/Predictions	Cognitive Distortions	Alternative Thoughts

Coping Statements

Sometimes you may feel so uncomfortable that you cannot even think of questions to help counter your negative thoughts. In this situation, you can try any of the following coping statements. Here are some examples:

- "I feel warm…so what?"
- "I'm just going to stick this out."
- "I'm just going to wait and let this pass."
- "This won't last forever."
- "I am not alone in this; there are others who understand what I am going through."

You can use any of these coping statements, or come up with some of your own. If you have catastrophic thoughts, you also can try saying *Don't even go there!* to yourself or the equivalent. These kinds of statements can help you balance your thoughts and find greater emotional equilibrium.

SUMMING IT ALL UP

- Hot flashes (sometimes called night sweats) are spontaneous episodes of heat dissipation that generate warmth or sweating that you usually feel on your chest, neck, and face due to the dilation of blood vessels just under your skin.

- Hot flashes usually last from one to five minutes and may be accompanied by other symptoms, such as increased heart rate and anxiety.

- Monitoring your hot flashes using a symptom diary can provide you with important information for managing this symptom by helping you understand the symptom in terms of its component parts: situational triggers, thoughts, feelings, and behaviors.

- Paced respiration and other behavioral strategies can be effective tools for reducing the impact of hot flashes. You won't know if a strategy works until you try it and see for yourself. Behavioral strategies can be simple yet powerful.

- Cognitive strategies can help you identify your thoughts, determine if they are distorted and distressing, and replace them with thoughts that are more realistic and helpful.

CHAPTER 6

Coping with Anxiety

What is anxiety?

What are the similarities between anxiety and a hot flash?

How could changing my thoughts help me cope with anxiety?

How could changing my behaviors help?

You have arrived at this chapter because you are experiencing more anxiety than usual. You may find your anxiety uncomfortable or even debilitating. There may be several reasons why you are experiencing more anxiety at this time, and you may or may not know what they are. Perhaps you have noticed that your anxiety level has increased since you started the menopausal transition. Maybe you are uncertain if the sudden increases in body temperature that you've been experiencing are the result of anxiety or if they are hot flashes. Or your hot flashes may be accompanied by anxiety, in that you fear people noticing.

Neither having a hot flash nor experiencing anxiety is very pleasant, and there is no doubt that one can often influence the other. For instance, the sudden escalation of body heat initiated by a hot flash can be intensified by the experience of anxiety. Or, if you start to feel anxious while preparing for an important work meeting, thinking *I have to really do well in front of all my colleagues*, your body's elevated temperature could potentially set off a hot flash. It can be difficult at times to disentangle the two.

Because there are many other reasons you may experience anxiety besides anticipating or having a hot flash, it is important to learn more about anxiety in general.

UNDERSTANDING ANXIETY

Anxiety is a normal emotion that everyone experiences from time to time. There are endless circumstances in which you may experience anxiety. Anxiety tends to be associated with negative or unpleasant events, such as waiting for the result of a loved one's surgery or getting stood up for a date, but anxiety in other circumstances can have a beneficial function. For example, anxiety might motivate you to prepare for a work evaluation, a test, or a performance.

What makes you anxious and how you react emotionally to those triggers depends on who you are. The specific symptoms of anxiety vary from person to person, as do their intensity and frequency.

When Anxiety Becomes Problematic

Anxiety becomes a problem when it interferes with your day-to-day functioning and causes you a lot of distress. This may happen if your anxiety is frequent or if you are greatly bothered by your symptoms and anxiety interferes with your life on a daily basis. If this is the case, you may be experiencing an anxiety disorder. This chapter will be helpful for you regardless of whether you have been diagnosed with an anxiety disorder, fear that you have one, or are experiencing a milder case of anxiety.

Anxiety disorders take many forms, from chronic, uncontrollable worries to intense episodes of physical symptoms that escalate into a panic attack. A panic attack is an unexpected rush of intense physical symptoms that may cause you to fear that you are having a heart attack, losing control, or even dying.

Even if not a diagnosable disorder, anxiety can cause problems. A common response to anxiety is avoidance of situations that trigger an anxious response. Avoidance works effectively in the short term to reduce your anxiety, but in the long term, avoidance significantly limits your life.

Treatments for Anxiety

Effective treatments for anxiety include CBT, medication, and a combination of CBT and medication. In this chapter, we will provide you with the basic cognitive behavioral strategies that have been proven effective in reducing the symptoms of anxiety. A significant amount of research has been done on managing anxiety. If you find that this chapter is not enough, or if you have suffered from an anxiety disorder before you began the menopausal transition, we recommend checking with your family doctor to access additional resources that you may need.

CHANGING HOW YOU SEE ANXIETY

The most important step in managing anxiety is to change how you view your experience of it. This can be done by breaking your experience down into its most basic elements: how you felt physically, what you thought, and what you did. These basic elements have been described as the three components of anxiety (Antony and Swinson 2000).

Think about a recent time that you felt intense anxiety. Did you notice any changes in your body? Was your heart racing? Did your temperature rise? These and other physical sensations are the *physiological* component of anxiety. What was going through your mind at the time you started to become anxious? Were you fearful that something negative would happen? Did images of this negative outcome appear in your mind? These types of mental experiences composed of thoughts or images are the *cognitive* component of anxiety. Finally, how did you react in that anxious situation? Did you leave abruptly? Perhaps once the anxiety started, you didn't even make it to where you were intending on going. These types of reactions are the *behavioral* component of anxiety.

Figure 6.1 shows the interactive nature of the three components of anxiety.

Physical Sensations
e.g., heart racing, feeling hot

Thoughts
e.g., predicting something bad will happen

Behaviors
e.g., escape or avoid situation

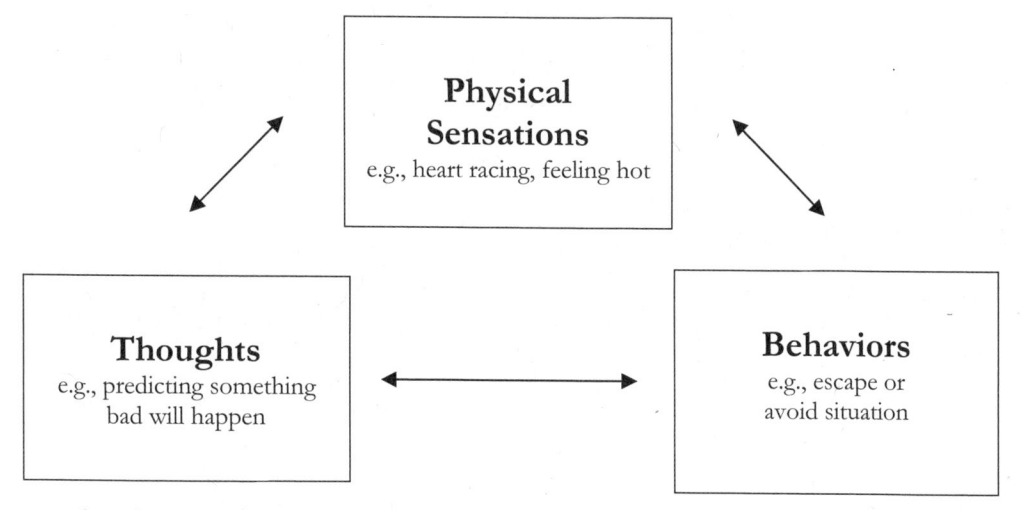

Figure 6.1: The three components of anxiety

As you see, this model for anxiety closely resembles the CBT model for how thoughts, feelings, behaviors, and physical sensations are connected. As the three components of anxiety interact with each other, your anxiety may increase or decrease in response to your thoughts and behaviors. Here is a closer look at each of the three components of anxiety.

The Physiological Component

The physiological component of anxiety is often the one that people notice when they first become anxious. It is all of the physical sensations that you experience:

- sweating
- dizziness
- feeling shaky
- heart racing or pounding
- dry mouth
- tingling or numbness in your hands or feet

- muscle weakness or stiffness
- blurred vision
- flushed face or neck
- tightness or pressure in your chest
- feeling short of breath or feeling smothered
- upset stomach or nausea

These physical sensations of anxiety can lead to anxious thoughts and behaviors.

The Cognitive Component

The cognitive component of anxiety includes worries, images, predictions, and beliefs, such as noticing changes in your heartbeat and interpreting the situation as dangerous. Some common examples of worry thoughts are:

- *I will never be able to get through this situation.*
- *This will end badly.*
- *Everyone will think that there is something wrong with me.*

Such worry thoughts will encourage anxious behaviors and increase your physical sensations of anxiety.

The Behavioral Component

The behavioral component of anxiety often includes reactions that seem helpful at the time but may end up actually prolonging your anxiety. These reactions include checking, escape, and avoidance.

Checking would include checking where the washroom is; checking your reflection for signs of physiological changes, such as sweating; checking your heart rate; checking to see if others are looking at you; and checking out all of the exits in the room you are in, so you can exit easily if need be. These behaviors may be helpful in the short term for reducing anxiety, but in the long run, they actually maintain your anxiety.

Escape is another common response. For example, when you are in a situation that is intensely anxiety provoking, you may feel as though you cannot tolerate it any longer, and so you leave sooner than intended. You may experience an immediate relief after leaving, but in the long term, this behavior encourages a habit of escaping or avoiding anxiety-provoking situations, which maintains rather than reduces your anxiety.

Avoidance is a common response that was mentioned earlier. You may feel so anxious about a situation that you simply choose not to attend or be involved. You avoid the event or choose not to put yourself in the situation at all. This is a natural response to extreme anxiety, and in the short term, it may be very effective at reducing your anxiety. However, in the long term, avoidance can lead to lower self-esteem, decreased confidence in your ability to cope, and in some cases an exaggerated dependence on other people.

Understanding how you tend to react to anxiety—in terms of how you physically feel, what you think, and how you behave—will help you manage your anxiety. Again, you can reduce your experience of anxiety by changing how you think and how you respond.

THE FACES OF ANXIETY

What causes anxiety will depend on who you are as an individual. Furthermore, your experience of anxiety—your physical sensations, your thoughts and predictions, and how you behave—will differ from someone else's. Here's a look at how two different women experienced anxiety.

▪ *Ellen's Story*

Ellen again began to experience anxiety attacks, also known as panic attacks, at the start of late perimenopause. She described experiencing increased body temperature, a racing heart, sweating, and dizziness. When Ellen noticed these physical sensations, she wondered whether it was a hot flash coming on or if it was something more. Her anxiety escalated, and she worried that something bad would happen, like she might faint.

One time, she experienced a panic attack when she suddenly developed a number of physical sensations while grocery shopping. She was so concerned that her symptoms were something other than the result of a hot flash or anxiety that she feared she might faint. Ellen abruptly left the store, abandoning her groceries in the cart. Now Ellen finds it very difficult to go to that grocery store for fear that she will have another panic attack there. She avoids grocery shopping by asking her husband to pick things up on his way home from work. Ellen also finds that she avoids other crowded shopping situations like the mall because of her concerns about having a panic attack.

Ellen's experience can be broken down into the three components of anxiety, as follows:

Physiological: Increased temperature, racing heart, sweating, dizziness.

Cognitive: *Something bad will happen. I will faint.*

Behavioral: Escape when she experiences these physical sensations and avoidance of grocery stores and shopping malls.

▪ *Jane's Story*

Jane noticed that she started to experience increased anxiety when her hot flashes became more unpredictable. For instance, while having an enjoyable conversation with friends at a dinner party, Jane's body sweating went into overdrive out of the blue. She started to become anxious with worry, wondering whether others would notice her hot flash. Her attention started to deviate from the conversation. She began to check her clothes to see if the sweat had come through. She also wondered if she was red in the face and excused herself to check in the bathroom mirror. Jane ended up leaving the party much earlier than she'd planned.

The next day, Jane had a lunch date with friends. On the way there, Jane started to fear that a hot flash would happen again and almost called to cancel at the last minute.

Jane's experience can be broken down into the three components of anxiety, as follows:

Physiological: Increased temperature, racing heart, sweating.

Cognitive: *Everyone will notice I am having a hot flash, and I will be embarrassed. There is something physically wrong with me. This is intolerable.*

Behavioral: Checking her clothes; checking her reflection; escaping by leaving earlier than planned; urge to avoid next social gathering.

Comparing Anxiety and Hot Flashes

It can be difficult to disentangle a hot flash from an anxiety-related experience, as both may involve an increase in your body temperature. Furthermore, as you can tell from Ellen's story, a hot flash may produce anxiety, and anxiety may increase the intensity of a hot flash. The sudden escalation of Ellen's body heat was initiated by a hot flash, but the physiological experience intensified as Ellen's anxiety escalated. Even wondering whether her increase in body temperature was a hot flash or a panic attack caused a further increase in body temperature, which in turn led to Ellen's anxiety increasing, as she worried that she was going to have a panic attack and faint. Figure 6.2 displays how similar the experiences of an anxiety attack and a hot flash can be.

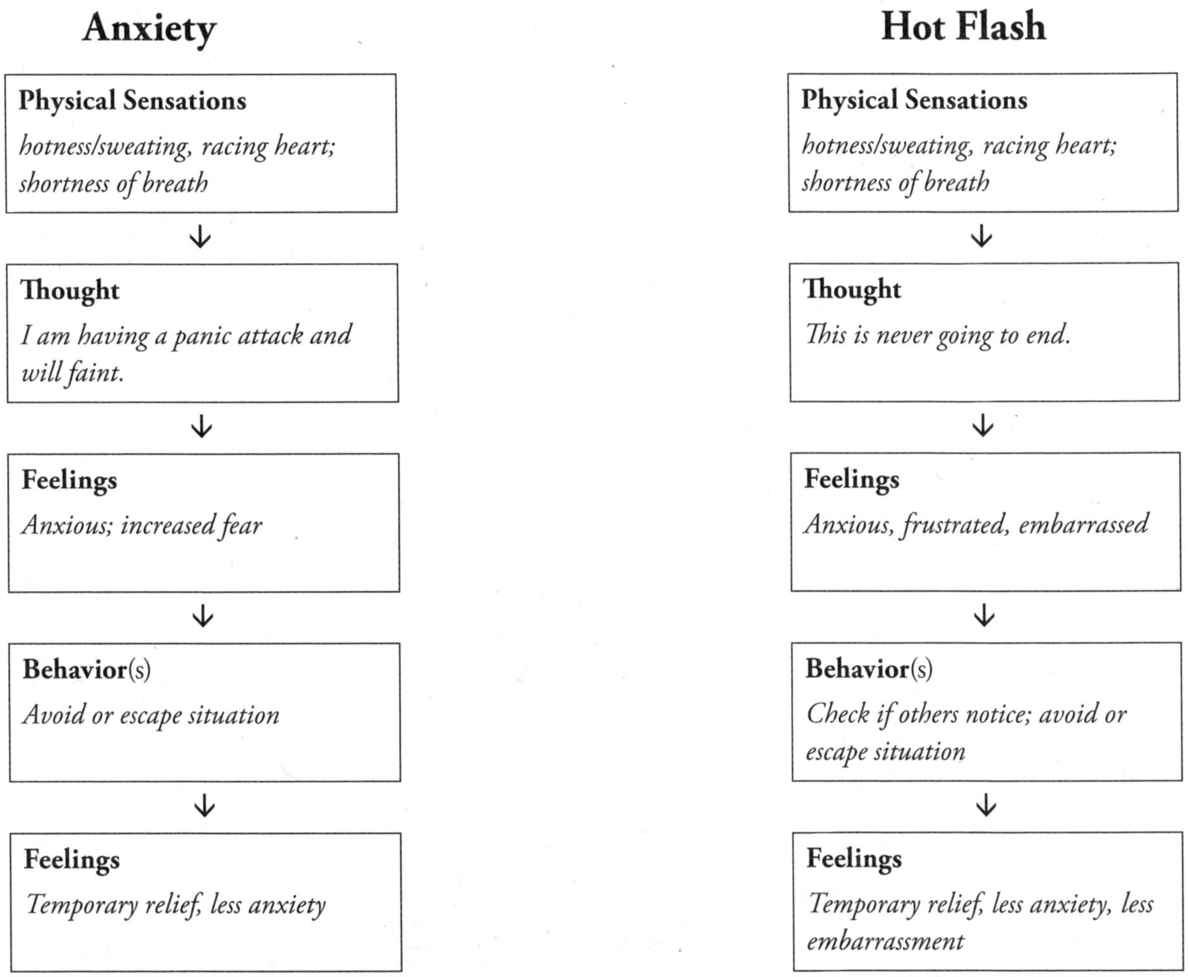

Coping with Anxiety

Anxiety

Physical Sensations
hotness/sweating, racing heart; shortness of breath

↓

Thought
I am having a panic attack and will faint.

↓

Feelings
Anxious; increased fear

↓

Behavior(s)
Avoid or escape situation

↓

Feelings
Temporary relief, less anxiety

Hot Flash

Physical Sensations
hotness/sweating, racing heart; shortness of breath

↓

Thought
This is never going to end.

↓

Feelings
Anxious, frustrated, embarrassed

↓

Behavior(s)
Check if others notice; avoid or escape situation

↓

Feelings
Temporary relief, less anxiety, less embarrassment

Figure 6.2: Anxiety vs. hot flash experience

As you can see, the physical trigger for anxiety is the same whether you're experiencing anxiety or a hot flash. No matter what causes it, the physical sensation of suddenly overheating is the trigger. Note that the components of these two experiences reflect the components of the CBT model, presented again in figure 6.3.

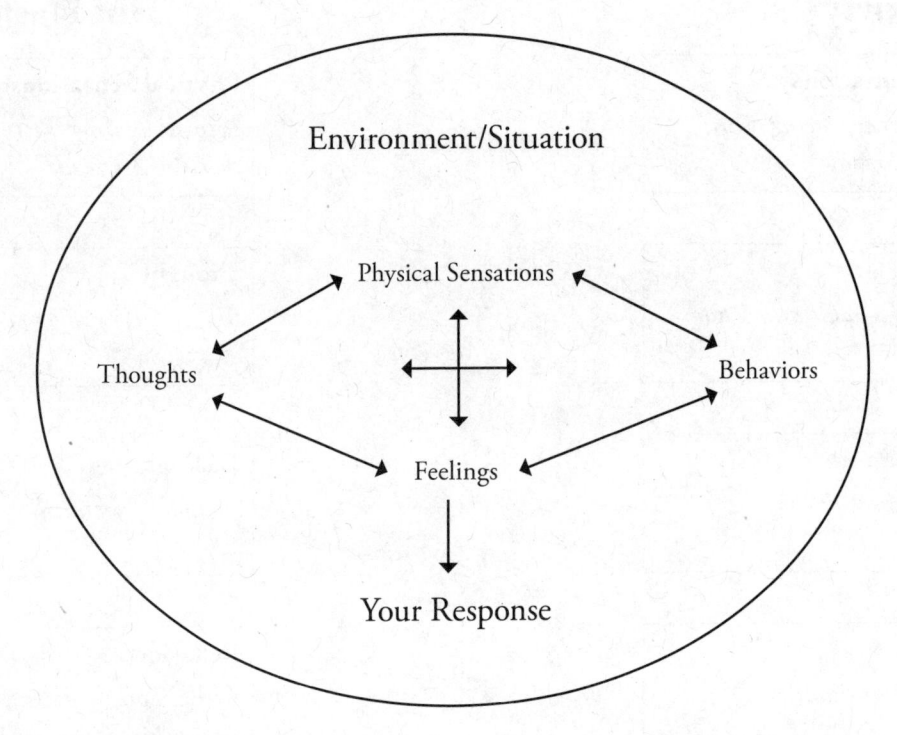

Figure 6.3: The CBT model

> # Quick Check
>
> If you were going to intervene with a strategy to feel better and reduce your anxiety or the intensity or distress of your hot flash, where would you do it on the CBT model in figure 6.3? What would you modify?
>
> 1. your experience/situation
> 2. your physical sensations
> 3. your thoughts
> 4. your feelings
> 5. your behavior
>
> **Answer:** The correct answer would be 3 and 5. You could intervene with a strategy to modify your thoughts (or how you interpret your physical sensations) and your behaviors. You cannot always control the situation or experience you find yourself in, your physical sensations, or your initial feelings or emotional response.

MONITORING YOUR EXPERIENCE

So what have you been experiencing? By monitoring your experiences more closely, you can break down your experience into multiple components that are consistent with the CBT model as well as the three components of anxiety. Doing this will give you more information about your experience and help you discover certain triggers and patterns, which will, in turn, help as you begin to apply cognitive and behavioral strategies to improve your experience.

The following anxiety monitoring form shows how Ellen and Jane monitored their experiences of anxiety.

Sample Anxiety Monitoring Form

Situation	Feelings (0–100)	Physical Sensations	Thoughts	Behaviors
Ellen: Sunday afternoon at the grocery store by myself shopping for groceries when I started to feel hot and noticed my heart racing.	anxious (80)	hot/sweating, racing heart, rapid breathing	Something bad will happen. I will faint.	Left the grocery store immediately, without any groceries.
Jane: At a friend's dinner party enjoying a conversation about my summer vacation with others, I started to feel hot.	embarrassed (80), distress (80), anxiety (70)	hot/sweating, racing heart	Everyone will notice I am having a hot flash. There is something physically wrong with me. This is intolerable.	Left the dinner party earlier than planned.

Your Anxiety Monitoring Form

Use the following anxiety monitoring form to record any experiences of anxiety that you have over the next week. Describe the situation you were in (what you were doing, whom you were with, and where you were), the feelings you had and their intensity on a scale of 0 to 100 (where 0 is the least intense and 100 is the most intense), what physical sensations you experienced (how your body reacted, what physical sensations increased), your thoughts (what was going through your mind before and after), and your behaviors (your response, what you did).

Situation	Feelings (0–100)	Physical Sensations	Thoughts	Behaviors

Reflecting on the Components of Anxiety

After monitoring your experiences of anxiety, you can reflect on this information to decide whether what you experienced was anxiety or a hot flash—or perhaps both anxiety and a hot flash—and to determine what strategies to try in order to manage your symptoms. To do this, you will need to take a step back and look for certain triggers, thoughts, and patterns. Here's what Ellen and Jane learned from this exercise.

Ellen's and Jane's Reflections

1. When do you tend to experience anxiety that is particularly distressing for you?

    Ellen: *At the grocery store and the mall.*

    Jane: *Usually around others in social situations, such as lunch with friends.*

2. What type of negative thoughts or predictions do you have when you experience anxiety?

    Ellen: *Something bad will happen, such as fainting.*

    Jane: *Others will see my hot flash and judge me in a negative way. They may think there is something wrong with me or think I am incompetent. They may think that I am anxious. Also, I find that the experience feels intolerable, like it is never going to end.*

3. What are you avoiding as a result of anxiety? What aspects of your life does your anxiety interfere with or disrupt? What kind of impact does this have on your quality of life?

    Ellen: *Grocery stores, any kind of shopping malls. This is very difficult for me as I need to shop for a number of things on a weekly basis. My family depends on me to get these tasks done, and I feel like a failure, but my anxiety is so great, I can't overcome it.*

    Jane: *I've found that I don't accept as many social invitations as I used to and I often cancel those that I do accept. This is a big deal for me, as I used to be so involved with my friends, and now I have isolated myself, which makes me feel depressed.*

4. How do the different components you have recorded (your thoughts, physical sensations, and behaviors) interact with each other to influence your level of anxiety?

    Ellen: *I noticed that as soon as I feel myself getting hot, I start to think that something bad is going to happen, like I could faint. This thought makes me feel very anxious and then I notice that my physical symptoms increase—my heart starts racing and I feel short of breath. When my physical symptoms increase, it feels like proof that something bad is really going to happen, so then I make a decision to leave.*

    Jane: *I notice that my concern that others will notice my hot flash seems to increase my focus on the physical symptoms that I have, and then they increase in intensity. The thought that it's never going to end makes me feel hopeless and influences my decision to leave a situation or avoid it altogether.*

Your Reflections

Based on your anxiety monitoring form, answer the following questions.

1. When do you tend to experience anxiety that is particularly distressing for you?

   _____
   _____
   _____

2. What type of negative thoughts or predictions do you have when you experience anxiety?

   _____
   _____
   _____

3. What are you avoiding as a result of anxiety? What aspects of your life does your anxiety interfere with or disrupt? What kind of impact does this have on your quality of life?

   _____
   _____
   _____

4. How do the different components you have recorded (your thoughts, physical sensations, and behaviors) interact with each other to influence your level of anxiety?

   _____
   _____
   _____

In this exercise, you've observed and monitored the components of your anxiety. This is important as it allowed you to step back from your intense physical experience of anxiety and analyze it. You may have noticed particular patterns among the situational triggers for your anxiety, your physical symptoms, your thoughts and interpretations, and your behavioral responses. You're now in a good position to learn some strategies for coping better with your anxiety and related physical distress.

COGNITIVE STRATEGIES FOR COPING WITH ANXIETY AND PHYSICAL DISTRESS

Now that you've monitored your experience with anxiety, you can focus on your thoughts and the impact that they have on your mood and behavior in various situations. Again, your thoughts, beliefs, and the way in which you interpret things can play an important role in how you experience life. They can have a negative impact on your mood by increasing your feelings of anxiety or depression, for example. As you may have noticed from analyzing your experience of anxiety, your thoughts also directly influence your behavior and the intensity of the physical sensations that you experience.

Thoughts that cause people to be anxious usually tend to focus on potential danger or harm in a situation as well as the inability to cope. For example, Jane was afraid people would notice her hot flash and think negatively of her, and she felt she couldn't tolerate the symptom. The goal with cognitive strategies is to identify your anxious thoughts, ask yourself whether they are realistic, and if they're not, consider a more realistic or balanced view of the situation. As you know from the CBT model, if you change one factor in your situation, you will affect all the other factors. Changing how you think about a situation will affect how you feel and cope. The more realistic your thought is, the less likely you are to feel anxious.

Some Common Cognitive Distortions

Two common cognitive distortions associated with anxiety are probability overestimation and catastrophizing (Barlow and Craske 1994).

PROBABILITY OVERESTIMATION

Probability overestimation involves thinking that a negative event is far more likely to occur than it actually is. The following two thoughts are examples of probability overestimation often associated with hot flashes and anxiety.

- *Whenever I have a hot flash, someone notices.*
- *If I start to feel hot or anxious, I could faint.*

When you are anxious, it often feels like the likelihood or probability of a bad outcome is very high. With this view, it then makes sense that your anxiety level will be high as well. Take Jane for example. When asked, she reported the probability of others noticing her hot flash as 100 percent. In fact, the realistic probability is much lower. When she disclosed to her close friend that she was embarrassed by her hot flash at the dinner party, her friend was completely surprised because she hadn't taken notice. If Jane were to focus more on the realistic probability of others noticing her hot flash, her anxiety would probably be lower.

Ellen also engages in probability overestimation in predicting that she will probably faint when she experiences hot flashes or high anxiety. In fact, Ellen has never actually fainted in her life. So the realistic probability of her passing out when she experiences a hot flash or panic attack is extremely low. Based on her past experience, it would be 0 percent likely.

When you are feeling anxious, do you find that you overestimate the likelihood of a negative outcome? If so, you are definitely not alone.

CATASTROPHIZING

Catastrophizing involves thinking that if a negative event actually did happen, it would be horrible or unbearable and impossible to cope with. Here are some examples of catastrophic thinking:

- *If I had a hot flash and someone noticed, it would be awful and humiliating.*

- *If I fainted in the grocery store, it would be the worst experience.*

These types of thoughts are distortions of reality because if the feared event (being noticed or fainting in the grocery store) were to happen, although unpleasant, the outcome would really not be that bad. Although people may notice Jane is sweating, would they really think horrible things about her? Realistically, most people probably wouldn't notice, and those who did might think she was just hot or that perhaps she was having a hot flash. They might actually feel bad for her discomfort. They would probably not think it was a big deal and would certainly prefer her to stay and be sweaty, so they could enjoy her company, rather than have her leave. Even if someone did think negatively of her, you could wonder, would this type of person be someone for whose opinion she should really care?

For Ellen, having a panic attack in the grocery store probably is a very unpleasant experience, but fainting in the grocery store is likely not the worst thing that could happen to her. People have been known to have medical emergencies in grocery stores, and the staff is trained to assist people who are in trouble and to call for medical help if needed. Although it might be embarrassing, it is unlikely that the shoppers would even remember Ellen on future visits if she did actually collapse in the store.

Taking the Three-Step Approach

You can use the three-step approach for shifting your thoughts to decrease your experiences of anxiety and associated physical distress. As you will recall from chapter 4, step one is to note your thoughts in a particular situation. You've already begun taking this step as you recorded your thoughts in the last exercise.

In step two, you identify your unhelpful thoughts or cognitive distortions. That is, you examine your thoughts to see if any represent examples of probability overestimation, catastrophizing, or any other cognitive distortions.

The final step is to consider ways of thinking about a situation that are more realistic or helpful. To help counter your anxious thoughts, you can ask yourself the following questions:

- "Based on my own experience, what is the realistic likelihood of this negative event happening?"

- "If this negative event did happen, how bad would it really be?"

Coping with Anxiety

- "What strengths and coping abilities do I have to help me manage this challenging situation?"

- "What advice for dealing with this situation would a close family member or friend give me?"

- "How would my close family member or friend handle this situation?"

- "What is the worst thing that could happen in this situation? How bad would it really be?"

- "Is this thought a realistic concern that I need to find a solution for?"

- "Is this a helpful way of looking at the situation? Is there another way of seeing things that would be more helpful?"

- "Are these thoughts my anxiety talking? If I weren't anxious, how would I think differently about this situation?"

You're now ready to start keeping a thought record, where you can record your thoughts, look for cognitive distortions, and counter your unhelpful or unrealistic thinking with alternative ways of viewing the situation.

Keeping a Thought Record

Keeping a thought record can help you begin to recognize and challenge any distorted thinking that's contributing to your experiences of anxiety or physical distress. As you practice countering your anxious thoughts, you may find it challenging to generate thoughts that are more realistic or helpful. The more you practice, however, the more skilled you will become. At first, you may find that anxious thoughts overpower your alternative thoughts, but this power balance will shift as you continue to practice countering your anxious thoughts. The following thought record shows how Ellen and Jane each did this exercise.

Sample Thought Record

Situation	Feelings (0–100)	Thoughts/ Predictions	Cognitive Distortions	Alternative Thoughts
Ellen: Sunday afternoon at the grocery store by myself shopping for groceries for the week	anxious (80)	Something bad will happen. I will faint.	probability overestimation catastrophizing	I have felt like this many times before and have never fainted. Although it feels 90 percent likely, realistically it is less than 1 percent likely. I am just having anxiety. I can cope with this and ride it out. These feelings will pass. They always do eventually. It is not pleasant, but I will feel better if I stick it out and finish my shopping.
Jane: At a good friend's dinner party enjoying a conversation about my summer vacation with others when I started to feel hot	embarrassed (80) distress (80) anxiety (70)	Everyone will notice I am having a hot flash. There is something physically wrong with me. This is intolerable.	probability overestimation (also mind reading) catastrophizing	People are probably not even noticing that I am sweating. Even if they are, they wouldn't be thinking negatively of me. These are my friends. They care about me. This is just a hot flash. It's unpleasant, but I can manage it. I can make a joke about it if someone says something. I know it will pass eventually. I will feel worse if I leave.

Now it's your turn to complete your thought record. Before you begin, you may want to make photocopies for future use or keep a thought record in a separate journal if you need more space.

Your Thought Record

Over the next week, use the following thought record three to five times to practice identifying your cognitive distortions and countering your anxious thoughts whenever you experience anxiety or panic. First describe the situation you were in (what you were doing, whom you were with, and where you were), the feelings you had and their intensity on a scale of 0 to 100 (where 0 is the least intense and 100 is the most intense), your thoughts and predictions (what was going through your mind before and after), the cognitive distortions behind these thoughts, and alternative thoughts to counter your unrealistic or unhelpful thinking. Use the list of questions to help you complete the alternative thoughts column.

Situation	Feelings (0–100)	Thoughts/Predictions	Cognitive Distortions	Alternative Thoughts

Any time you feel anxious, you can use the thought record to challenge your thoughts. Eventually, you will find that this skill becomes so automatic that you will not even need a thought record. You will be able to counter an anxious thought as soon as it pops into your mind.

BEHAVIORAL STRATEGIES FOR COPING WITH ANXIETY

The three-step cognitive approach you have learned is a powerful technique for changing both how you feel and what you do in response to anxiety. You can also change how you feel and how you think by directly targeting your behavior. The behaviors associated with anxiety that you will want to target are checking, escape, and avoidance. All of these behaviors serve to maintain and even increase your anxiety.

Checking

When you are anxious, you may become hypervigilant to what's going on around you, as well as to changes happening inside your body, in an attempt to be alert to possible threats or danger. To eliminate checking behaviors, you can catch yourself monitoring these things and mentally step back from the situation. Whether you are monitoring your body for symptoms, your environment for exits, or other people's reactions to you, you will want to shift your focus to whatever activity you are participating in. For example, Jane might shift the focus of her attention away from monitoring her body and other people's reactions and instead focus on the conversation going on around her. You can use the cognitive strategies you have learned to help you address an anxious thought directly and then consciously shift the focus of your attention.

The Urge to Escape

When you feel anxious, the urge to escape a situation that you perceive as dangerous makes sense biologically. It's a protective response in the face of real danger. But when no danger is present, choosing to escape can be counterproductive, especially over time. While escaping a situation can be powerfully effective for reducing your anxiety in the short term, such as when you feel anxious in a party full of strangers and choose to leave the party, responding this way in the long term allows your anxiety to take control of your life, such as when you begin turning down social invitations if you think you might have a hot flash and begin to panic.

When you are faced with an urge to escape a situation, you can use the three-step cognitive approach to address your anxious thoughts head on. If you encourage yourself to tolerate your anxiety, especially the physical sensations, it will eventually pass. The more practice you have in riding out your anxiety, the more confident you will become, knowing that you can do anything in spite of your anxiety. Remind yourself of how good you will feel if you stay in a situation that you know is safe, even as your anxiety is making you feel like you want to escape.

Avoidance

Your anxiety may have become so powerful that you are avoiding situations that trigger it. The more situations that you avoid, the greater the impact anxiety has on your ability to function and your quality of life.

The main strategy for targeting avoidance is situational exposure, which involves gradually confronting the situations you are avoiding in a step-by-step approach. Practicing exposure will allay your fears as you realize through this process that there was nothing to be afraid of after all.

Coping with Anxiety

The first step is to make a list of the situations you are avoiding because of your anxiety and rate how anxious you would be in each of these situations. The next step is to reorganize the list starting with the most anxiety-provoking situation and ending with the least anxiety-provoking situation. This is called an *exposure hierarchy*, which ranks your fears in order from greatest to least. Ellen's exposure hierarchy is an example of this sort of list.

Ellen's Exposure Hierarchy

	Situation	Anxiety Level (0–100)
1.	Going to shopping mall by myself when it is crowded.	95
2.	Going to grocery store by myself when it is crowded.	90
3.	Going to shopping mall with a friend when it is crowded.	85
4.	Driving on the highway by myself in heavy traffic.	80
5.	Going to grocery store with a friend when it is crowded.	80
6.	Driving on the highway with a friend in heavy traffic.	75
7.	Going to shopping mall by myself when it is not crowded.	70
8.	Going to grocery store by myself when it is not crowded.	65
9.	Driving on the highway by myself in light traffic.	60
10.	Going to convenience store.	50
11.	Waiting in line at the bank.	40
12.	Driving on the highway with a friend when there is light traffic.	30

You can see that Ellen typically avoids twelve situations, including going to shopping malls, stores, and driving on the highway. Different factors increase or decrease her anxiety level in these situations, including whether she is alone or with a close friend, whether a store is crowded or not, and how heavy traffic is. Her exposure hierarchy is organized from most anxiety-provoking situation to least.

Situations You Avoid Due to Anxiety

List all the situations you avoid due to fear of anxiety. Include any factors that might significantly change your anxiety level in a situation, such as whether you are alone or with a friend. Next, review each situation on the list and record how anxious you would feel in that situation, rating your anxiety on a scale of 0 to 100, where 0 represents the least anxiety and 100 represents the most anxiety you might feel.

Situation	Anxiety Level (0–100)

The next step is to reorganize your list as an exposure hierarchy, which you can then use as a basis for practicing exposure to the situations that you usually avoid.

Your Exposure Hierarchy

Look at the list of situations that you avoid because of anxiety, and list the situations again, this time in order from most anxiety-provoking (the situation that you most want to avoid) to least anxiety-provoking. List the anxiety level that you associate with each situation, as you did before.

	Situation	Anxiety Level (0–100)
1.		
2.		
3.		
4.		
5.		
6.		
7.		
8.		
9.		
10.		

Practicing Exposure

Once you have completed your exposure hierarchy, you can begin practicing confronting the situations that you avoid. This is a gradual approach to confronting your fears in that you typically start with the least anxiety-provoking situation first, such as a situation that evokes an anxiety level of 30 or 40, although you can decide to start anywhere on your hierarchy.

The goal is to practice exposing yourself to the situation repeatedly until your anxiety is reduced by at least half. So if one situation provokes an anxiety level of 40 to begin with, you continue to expose yourself to that situation until your anxiety level is reduced to 20 for most of the time you're in that situation. Once this happens, you can move up your hierarchy to confront a situation that you associate with a higher level of anxiety. After your anxiety in that situation is reduced by at least half, you can move up the hierarchy again, and so on, until you have nothing left to fear.

It's best to go at a comfortable pace as you work your way up your hierarchy. You may want to practice with a friend at first, too, if doing so will help you confront a difficult fear. As you practice your exposures, you will find yourself becoming more comfortable and confident in managing the situations that trigger your anxiety. You can also use your cognitive strategies to help you confront any anxious thoughts that arise during exposure practice, since you will probably feel anxious at times as you engage in exposure. Although your anxiety may be temporarily increased in the short term, exposure is an extremely powerful technique for minimizing anxiety in the long term.

We recommend that you aim for daily exposure practice with one or two situations you have chosen to work on. If daily exposure is not practical, then try to complete a minimum of three practices per week. It will help to keep track of your exposure experience, as Ellen did using the following exposure practice form.

Ellen's Exposure Practice Form

Situation: *Drive on the highway by myself in light traffic.*

Initial anxiety level (0–100): *60*

Anxious thoughts: *I will have a panic attack. I will not be able to focus on my driving. I will have an accident.*

Countering thoughts: *I have driven many times when I have had a panic attack. Even though it feels terrible, I was able to focus and drive safely. The panic attack eventually passed. I know that a panic attack isn't dangerous. It just feels really horrible. I will feel better after this exposure practice because I am taking control back from the anxiety. I can do this.*

Length of exposure (minutes): *30 minutes*

Anxiety level (0–100) at end of exposure: *30*

What did you learn from this experience? *I was able to do it even though I felt anxious. Just because I feel that something bad will happen doesn't mean it will. Challenging my anxiety makes me feel better and more in control of my life—like I have regained a little bit of myself the way I was before the anxiety took over.*

Next exposure practice: *I will repeat this one again tomorrow.*

You should record your experience each time you conduct an exposure. Recording your experience will help you incorporate the cognitive strategies that you've learned, highlight important aspects of your experience, and monitor your progress in confronting your fears. Before you begin, you may want to make photocopies of the following blank form for later use.

Your Exposure Practice Form

Record the situation you are confronting and the anxiety level that you associate with it (see your exposure hierarchy). Write down your anxious thoughts and some countering thoughts that will help you confront your fears. Time the length of your exposure and record the time. At the end of the exposure, check your anxiety level. Is it lower than it was before exposure? On a scale of 0 to 100, where 0 represents the least and 100 the highest anxiety, what is your anxiety level after exposure? Next, record what you learned from this experience. Finally, write down when you will practice your next exposure.

Situation: _____

Initial anxiety level (0–100): _____

Anxious thoughts: _____

_____

_____

Countering thoughts: _____

_____

_____

Length of exposure (minutes): _____

Anxiety level (0–100) at end of exposure: _____

What did you learn from this experience? _____

_____

_____

Next exposure practice: _____

KEEPING YOUR ANXIETY IN CHECK

In this chapter, you learned the CBT strategies for tackling your anxiety. Now it is all about putting them into practice. As you continue to practice countering your anxious thoughts and challenging your anxiety through situational exposure, you will see your anxiety greatly reduce, and you will also start to feel more comfortable and confident in your ability to cope. If you do not see improvements, it may be that you need more specialized treatment. Your family doctor can assess your symptoms and make treatment recommendations, such as seeing a psychologist who is trained in treating anxiety.

SUMMING IT ALL UP

- During the menopausal transition, you may experience anxiety symptoms that significantly interfere with your quality of life and your day-to-day functioning.

- Anxiety can be broken down into three components that influence each other: thoughts, physical sensations, and behavior.

- Cognitive strategies can help you shift your anxious thoughts so that you are able to view a situation from a more helpful or realistic perspective.

- Behavioral strategies can target behaviors, such as checking, escape, and avoidance, that maintain and exacerbate your anxiety.

- If you find that your anxiety does not improve, your family doctor can assess your symptoms and determine the best treatment options for you.

CHAPTER 7

Dealing with Depression and Other Feelings

How common are depression and other mood-related difficulties during menopause?

What are the causes and risk factors of mood disturbances during this time?

What stressors and life changes may be influencing my mood?

What behavioral strategies can I use to improve my mood?

What cognitive strategies can I use?

The focus of this chapter is on the mood changes you may be experiencing during menopause. Although a number of challenges during this transition can have a negative impact on your life, most women will not experience clinical depression. But for those who do suffer from depression, cognitive behavioral therapy has been shown to be very effective. CBT strategies can also help you deal with mood changes during menopause even if you are not clinically depressed.

This chapter will help you identify and address the specific mood changes that concern you. It will explain how different factors, such as thoughts, behaviors, and life circumstances and stressors, can affect your mood, and it will show you how to use specific cognitive and behavioral strategies to help reduce the intensity and impact of your mood changes. This chapter will also help you determine if you may be experiencing clinical depression and whether you should seek additional help from your family doctor. First, here are some basic facts about depression during menopause.

DEPRESSION DURING MENOPAUSE

The term *depression* is used so widely, it can mean different things in terms of severity. For instance, when the average person states that he or she feels depressed, it usually refers to a brief period of feeling blue or sad. Different life events or circumstances, such as the loss of a job or a divorce, can cause feelings of sadness. Such periods of sadness are usually short and often do not require treatment, although if felt for a prolonged period, sad feelings can progress into a clinical depression. A clinical depression is when you consistently feel depressed for most of the day nearly every day for a minimum of two weeks, in addition to experiencing a number of other symptoms, such as loss of interest or pleasure in things you used to enjoy, poor concentration, difficulties with sleep, feelings of worthlessness, restlessness or lethargy, changes in appetite, and low energy (American Psychiatric Association 2000).

The menopausal transition can be a time of heightened risk for women to develop impairing depressive symptoms or even clinical depression. In particular, perimenopause is associated with the occurrence of depression in midlife women (Cohen et al. 2006).

Causes of Depression

There appears to be a complex relationship between hot flashes and depression (Joffe, Soares, and Cohen 2003), with some studies suggesting that severe vasomotor symptoms (such as hot flashes or night sweats) represent a red flag and indicate a heightened risk for the emergence or worsening of depressive symptoms. However, depression at this time in life can also occur independently of hot flashes. In some cases, it might be quite difficult for women and their doctors to determine whether depression is caused or triggered by hot flashes, sleep disturbances, hormonal changes, environmental stressors, thoughts, or other triggers that occur for women during menopause.

There are a few theories as to the cause of depression during menopause. For instance, the stress related to the management of menopausal symptoms has been thought to increase the risk for depression. In this case, women might find it too difficult to manage their menopausal symptoms in addition to other stressors in their life (such as new social roles, aging parents, or other medical conditions) at this time (Soares 2010).

Another proposed theory associates menopausal depression with fluctuating hormone levels. Levels of estrogen, progesterone, and androgen are constantly changing during menopause. These hormones are believed to influence areas in your brain that are crucial for mood regulation. With abrupt changes in hormones such as estrogen, you can experience a disruption in mood regulation, resulting in sadness and depression (Lokuge et al. 2011).

Risk Factors

In general, women are twice as likely as men to develop depression (Kessler et al. 2005). If you have a history of depression, you are more likely to develop depression during menopause. However, 26 to 33 percent of women will develop a first episode of depression during the menopausal transition, especially when there are a number of negative life stressors occurring at the same time (Cohen et al. 2006). Women who have experienced depression in the past associated with hormone changes (for example, during premenstrual or postpartum periods) and women who have gone through surgical menopause are also at increased risk for depression (Soares and Zitek 2008). In addition, being a smoker, having other medical conditions, and experiencing a number of psychosocial stressors are also associated with increased risk for developing depression during menopause (Frey, Lord, and Soares 2008).

Treatments for Depression

There are a number of very effective treatment options available for depression. Many antidepressants have been shown to be helpful for treating menopausal depression (Soares and Frey 2010).

Estrogen therapy, long used to alleviate hot flashes or night sweats, has recently shown good results in reducing symptoms of depression in perimenopausal and early postmenopausal women (Soares and Frey 2010). Its use is based on the theory that decreased or fluctuating levels of estrogen during menopause can trigger a depressive episode. Estrogen therapy may therefore be used not only to improve vasomotor symptoms but also to minimize hormonal changes and stabilize your mood. If you are interested in finding out more about these hormonal and nonhormonal treatment options and whether they are right for you, you should speak with your family physician or health care professional.

Psychotherapy, in particular CBT, has been shown to be very helpful on its own or combined with medical treatments to reduce menopause-associated depressive symptoms (Green et al. 2010). This chapter will present the CBT strategies typically used in treating depression. If you believe you have clinical depression, you should also seek help from your family physician.

Quick Check

Are you experiencing any of the following symptoms of clinical depression? Clinical depression is defined as follows (American Psychiatric Association 2000):

- ☐ feeling depressed every day, for most of the day, for at least a two-week period

or

- ☐ loss of interest or pleasure in things you usually enjoy (such as relationships or hobbies) for at least a two-week period

plus four of the following:

- ☐ loss of appetite or increased appetite accompanied by a significant weight loss or gain, such as ten pounds
- ☐ increased sleep (hypersomnia), or decreased or impaired sleep (insomnia)
- ☐ change in psychomotor activity, such as lethargy or agitation
- ☐ increased fatigue
- ☐ difficulty concentrating or making decisions
- ☐ excessive feelings of guilt or worthlessness
- ☐ suicidal thoughts

If at any time you experience suicidal thoughts or ideation, you should contact your health care provider or go to your nearest hospital emergency room.

In addition to feeling depressed, you may experience other feelings or emotions during the menopausal transition that can also be quite disruptive. Take a moment to consider whether you can relate to any of the following feelings:

Dealing with Depression and Other Feelings

- sad
- down
- irritable
- annoyed
- overwhelmed
- guilty
- lonely
- regretful
- stressed
- hopeless
- despairing
- unhappy
- impatient
- agitated

ENVIRONMENTAL INFLUENCES

Every phase of life has common stressors associated with it. These stressors may be related either to the *environment* or to the *situation* in the CBT model (figure 4.1). In childhood and adolescence, for example, common experiences that have the potential to turn into stressors include starting school, making friends, negotiating rules and expectations with your parents, going through puberty, and starting to date. In young adulthood, you probably crossed a number of bridges that could have increased your level of stress, such as figuring out what to do following high school, moving away from home, starting a career, or developing intimate relationships and getting married. Other common stressors prior to midlife include having and raising children, working hectic hours, coordinating the activities of each family member in a household, and trying to make ends meet.

There will always be stressors that accompany whatever phase in life that you are in. If you are a mother, you may no longer have the stress of raising young children at this time and might find that you are more financially secure as well. However, you may now be faced with the challenges of helping your children through adolescence or having your children move away from home, or perhaps you are about to become a grandparent or are considering retirement. Other stressors may include dealing with emerging health issues related to your aging parents. These life events can ultimately affect how you feel, what you think, and how you react.

The following circumstances, which are common during menopause, have the potential to become stressors:

- children growing up, becoming more independent, spending less time with the family, and even moving out or away (empty nest syndrome)
- additional family responsibilities, such as caring for an elderly parent
- transitioning from being able to physically have children to the loss of this ability
- retirement
- aging and considering the meaning and purpose of your life
- increased financial obligations with children in college, living away from home
- medical issues associated with the aging process (either yours or your loved ones')
- continued demands of juggling various responsibilities at work or home

The following exercise will help you look at some of the stressors that may be having an impact on your mood.

What Are the Stressors in Your Life?

Look over the list of stressors common to this time of life and write down any that apply to your experience. Add any other stressors that you can think of that may be influencing your mood.

1. _____

2. _____

3. _____

4. _____

Dealing with Depression and Other Feelings

Keep your list of identified life stressors in mind as you move forward.

Stressful Impacts

The CBT model, presented again in figure 7.1, shows how changes in your environment or situation may have a stressful impact on your feelings, thoughts, and behaviors.

```
                    Environment/Situation

                      Physical Sensations
                    ↗        ↕        ↖
            Thoughts  ←→    ↔       ←→  Behaviors
                    ↘        ↕        ↙
                          Feelings
                             ↓
                       Your Response
```

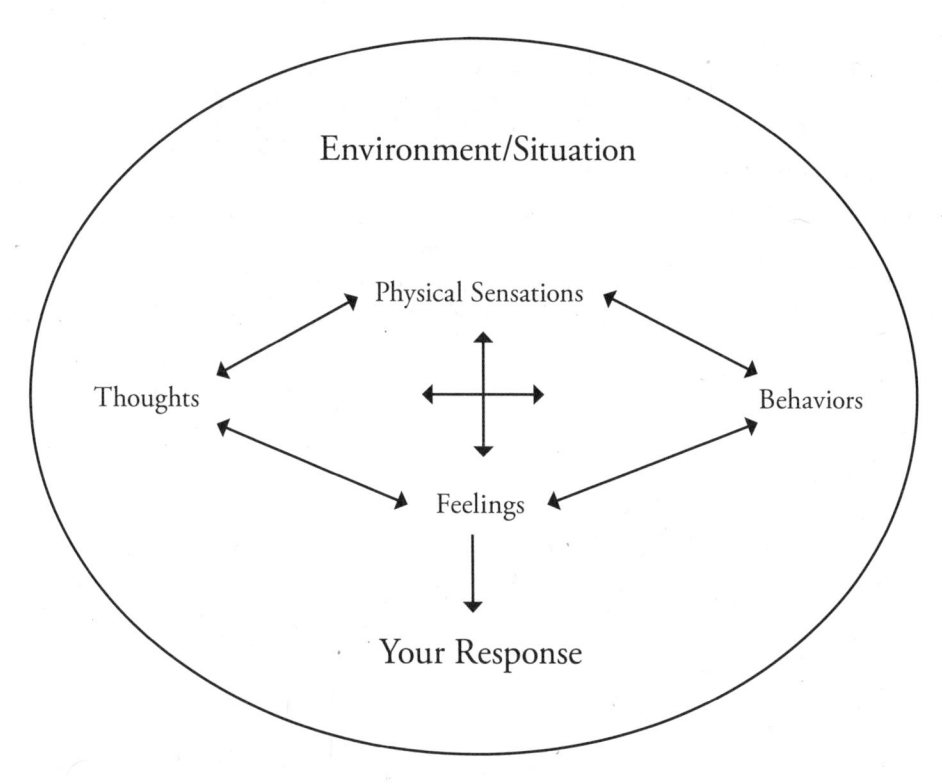

Figure 7.1: The CBT model

As one example, when your children leave home (changing circumstances in your environment or situation), you may begin to think *My children no longer need me*, you may feel depressed, and you may begin to withdraw and avoid social activities.

Environment/situation ⟶ **Feelings** (depression, despair)
(children moving out of family home)
                                Behaviors (withdraw, avoid)

                                Thought (*My children no longer need me.*)

As you are probably aware, it may not be possible to simply isolate or eliminate stressors in your life. For instance, though you may find it difficult when your children move out of the family home or when you are caring for an elderly parent, these circumstances cannot be easily changed. What you can do, however, is examine your thoughts, beliefs, behaviors, or reactions to these circumstances, figure out if they are problematic, and if so, change them, which in turn has the potential to ultimately change how you feel.

BEHAVIORAL INFLUENCES

Not only do environmental factors affect how you feel, but your behaviors do as well. By modifying your behaviors, you can change how you feel, but to do this, you must figure out what behaviors are contributing to your negative feelings. You can do this by monitoring your activities and rating how you feel as you engage in each activity. This will help you know if certain times of day are better or worse for you, help you become aware of how you feel at these times, and help you identify the reasons you feel this way.

The following monitoring form shows how Catherine kept a diary of her weekly activities and feelings. Catherine suffers from depression, so her feeling of depression was what she chose to monitor. Catherine rated these feelings on a 0 to 100 scale, where 0 represented when she felt the least depressed and 100 represented when she felt the most depressed.

Catherine's Weekly Activity and Feeling Monitoring Form

	Monday	Tuesday	Wednesday	Thursday	Friday	Saturday	Sunday
8:00 a.m.	Ready for work-50	Awake in bed-75	Ready for work-50	Awake in bed-75	Ready for work-50	Awake in bed-75	Awake in bed-75
9:00 a.m.	Start teaching-20	Awake in bed-75	Start teaching-20	Awake in bed-75	Start teaching-20	Awake in bed-75	Awake in bed-75
10:00 a.m.	Teaching-20	Awake in bed-75	Teaching-20	Awake in bed-75	Teaching-20	Awake in bed-75	Awake in bed-75
11:00 a.m.	Teaching-20	Ready for day-50	Teaching-20	Ready for day-50	Teaching-20	Ready for day-50	Ready for day-50
noon	Lunch staff room-20	Lunch with brother-10	Lunch staff room-90	Lunch-20	Lunch staff room-20	Lunch with friend-10	Cook for family dinner-20
1:00 p.m.	Teaching-20	Drive and prep-10	Teaching-20	Drive and prep-10	Teaching-20	Grocery shopping-25	Drive to parents' home-20
2:00 p.m.	Teaching-20	Special Ed-0	Teaching-20	Special Ed-0	Teaching-20	Cleaning house-50	Play with niece and nephew-10

Dealing with Depression and Other Feelings

	Monday	Tuesday	Wednesday	Thursday	Friday	Saturday	Sunday
3:00 p.m.	Teaching-20	Special Ed-0	Teaching-20	Special Ed-0	Teaching-20	Phone call friend-70	Play with niece and nephew-10
4:00 p.m.	Prepare dinner-25	Prepare dinner-25	Prepare dinner-25	Prepare dinner-25	Prepare dinner-20	Take out dinner alone-75	Dinner with family-10
5:00 p.m.	Dinner by self-75	Dinner by self-75	Dinner by self-75	Dinner by self-75	Dinner by self-75	TV-70	Dinner with family-10
6:00 p.m.	TV-60	TV-60	TV-60	TV-60	TV-60	TV-80	Dinner with family-10
7:00 p.m.	TV-60	Prep for teaching-20	TV-60	Yoga class-25	TV-60	TV-80	Clean for week-30
8:00 p.m.	TV-60	Prep for teaching-20	TV-60	Tidy home-25	TV-60	TV-80	Clean for week-30
9:00 p.m.	E-mail friends-10	Teaching prep-20	TV-60	Teaching prep-20	TV-60	TV-80	Make lunch-30
10:00 p.m.	Sleep-0	Sleep-0	Sleep-0	Sleep-0	Sleep-0	Sleep-0	Sleep-0
11:00 p.m.	Sleep-0	Sleep-0	Sleep-0	Sleep-0	Sleep-0	Sleep-0	Sleep-0

Over the next two weeks, you can use the following form to keep a record of your activities and the feeling that you want to monitor. Before you get started, you will need to make at least one photocopy.

Your Weekly Activity and Feeling Monitoring Form

Choose a feeling that you want to monitor over the next two weeks. You may choose to monitor depression or any other feeling—such as sad, down, irritable, annoyed, overwhelmed, guilty, lonely, regretful, stressed, hopeless, despairing, unhappy, impatient, or agitated—that you have identified as problematic in your life.

Keep track of what you do each hour of the day, and rate how much you experienced this feeling while you were doing each activity. Use a 0 to 100 scale, so that if you rate the feeling that you have chosen to monitor as a 0, this means that this particular feeling was not present during that hour. If you rate the feeling as 100, this means that the feeling was as intense as you have ever experienced it. When describing an activity for the hour and considering what to write, please simply record whatever you were doing; it may oftentimes be as straightforward as "phone call" or "grocery store."

	Monday	Tuesday	Wednesday	Thursday	Friday	Saturday	Sunday
8:00 a.m.							
9:00 a.m.							
10:00 a.m.							
11:00 a.m.							
noon							
1:00 p.m.							
2:00 p.m.							
3:00 p.m.							

Dealing with Depression and Other Feelings

4:00 p.m.	5:00 p.m.	6:00 p.m.	7:00 p.m.	8:00 p.m.	9:00 p.m.	10:00 p.m.	11:00 p.m.

Analyzing the Activity and Feeling Monitoring Form

After you've collected this information, you can probably recognize certain patterns of behavior, which will help guide your strategies in managing your depressive symptoms. Here is what Catherine learned from this exercise.

Catherine's Analysis of Her Activity and Feeling Monitoring Form

1. Were certain times of day more distressing for you than others? If yes, which ones, and why do you think these times of day were more distressing?

   As I examined my activity-feeling monitoring form I realized that although it felt like I was depressed all day, there were different times of day that were worse than others on a regular basis. Mornings are particularly challenging, especially when I tend to stay in bed and don't have anything scheduled like teaching. I also discovered that dinners alone and evenings are difficult for me. It seems like those times of the day, when I am not busy or I am alone, I tend to think a lot, and those thoughts tend to be depressing. Being alone never really bothered me before, but it seems since I entered into this stage in my life, I have been starting to question decisions I made in the past, and this has caused me to feel upset and unsure.

2. Were there certain times of day when you felt better than other times? If yes, which times were they and why do you think you felt better then?

   Whenever I am involved in an activity, my mood tends to be less intense. I did not think that I was getting much from it anymore, but teaching continues to be something I enjoy, and the specialized training I recently engaged in to teach special education to a disabled population is incredibly fulfilling for me. This is very reinforcing too, as I approach retirement within my regular teaching role and am faced with the question of how to spend my time and energy going forward. I also noticed how important my family life is to me. Seeing my parents, siblings, and nieces and nephews during Sunday dinner is such a special time and makes me think about planning to spend more time with them and be a part of the activities they are involved in.

3. Were there specific circumstances or activities that you engaged in when you noticed that your negative feelings quickly intensified?

   When I was in the staff room over lunch last Wednesday, a fellow staff member was discussing her daughter's upcoming wedding while another staff member was showing pictures of her new grandchild. My mood immediately plummeted, and I had to leave the room so that my colleagues did not see my tears. Moreover, I found myself tearing up while on the phone with a close friend on Saturday afternoon when she told me that she has decided to travel with her husband over the next year. Lately I have been questioning my choices in life. With menopause arriving, it is finally sinking in—my decision not to have children—and I wonder if I made a mistake. I also feel a bit of despair that I will never find a companion to spend my life with.

4. Overall, what are the patterns in your experience? Where do you think it might be helpful to intervene based on this information?

   Mornings are definitely very challenging. Times when I have meals by myself and evenings (when I am not doing anything) can also be difficult. These are the areas that need improvement.

The Cognitive Behavioral Workbook for Menopause

Your Analysis of Your Activity and Feeling Monitoring Form

Review what you wrote over the previous two weeks in your activity and feeling monitoring form, and answer the following questions.

1. Were certain times of day more distressing for you than others? If yes, which ones, and why do you think these times of day were more distressing?

   _____
   _____
   _____
   _____

2. Were there certain times of day when you felt better than other times? If yes, which times were they and why do you think you felt better then?

   _____
   _____
   _____
   _____

3. Were there specific circumstances or activities that you engaged in when you noticed that your negative feelings quickly intensified?

   _____
   _____
   _____
   _____

4. Overall, what are the patterns in your experience? Where do you think it might be helpful to intervene based on this information?

_____

_____

_____

_____

BEHAVIORAL STRATEGIES FOR CHANGING HOW YOU FEEL

One of the easiest and most straightforward ways of changing how you feel is through behavioral activation (Jacobson et al. 1996). *Behavioral activation*, as the name suggests, means getting active. One of the most problematic behaviors when you feel depressed is to either avoid activities or withdraw from them, particularly those that used to bring a sense of pleasure, enjoyment, or satisfaction.

Avoidance and withdrawal can be partially explained by the lack of energy that comes along with depression. In other words, you can simply feel too tired to attend a lunch date, even when it's something you would usually find enjoyable. Another reason is that you might not be getting the same amount of pleasure or enjoyment out of your usual activities, so you might feel unengaged and think to yourself, *Why bother if I do not enjoy it as much as I used to?* Further, you may find yourself believing that these activities will bring you no pleasure at all, given that you are feeling depressed. Whatever your reason for resisting it, activation is the key strategy to reduce isolation and avoid perpetuating depressive symptoms.

Choosing What to Do

That stated, it's never a good idea to just start doing random activities. In this case, one size does not fit all. For instance, gardening might be very pleasurable for some women and promote happiness and joy, while others might dislike working in the yard. Therefore, it is important to be strategic and engage in activities that give you pleasure or a sense of satisfaction or accomplishment. Some activities may give you both. The first step is to identify these activities, which you can do using the following worksheet.

Pleasurable or Enjoyable Activities

Take some time to make a list of activities that you have enjoyed in the past or that continue to bring you pleasure.

Dealing with Depression and Other Feelings

Activities That Bring a Sense of Satisfaction or Accomplishment

List activities that you do not necessarily enjoy but that give you a sense of satisfaction or a feeling that you have accomplished something. For instance, although you may not enjoy cleaning your home, it may give you a sense of satisfaction after you've done it.

_____   _____   _____

_____   _____   _____

_____   _____   _____

_____   _____   _____

_____   _____   _____

_____   _____   _____

_____   _____   _____

_____   _____   _____

_____   _____   _____

_____   _____   _____

Taking Action

The next step is to start engaging in some of these activities by strategically inserting them into your day. From monitoring your activities and feelings, you probably know where adding an activity might improve your mood. For example, Catherine's most challenging times are mornings when she is not working. She tends to stay in bed for a long time during these mornings. Thus, it would be ideal for Catherine to strategically add an enjoyable activity in the morning, such as taking a yoga class, to see if it has a positive impact on how she feels.

It is imperative to give any strategy a fair shot, which means not discarding the activity after one unsuccessful attempt but trying it out a few times to see if doing it really has a positive impact or not. You can use the following worksheet to track the success of trying out new activities over the next two weeks. Before you get started, you may want to make photocopies of the empty worksheet so that you can use it multiple times.

Expected Vs. Actual Pleasure/Satisfaction Record

Over the next two weeks, enter the time and date when you will do an activity that you've chosen to try out. Using a scale of 0 to 100, with 0 representing no pleasure and 100 representing the most pleasure, record the degree of pleasure you expect to experience before doing an activity and then record the degree of pleasure you actually experienced while performing it. Add your comments at the end of doing the activity each time you do it.

Date and Time	Activity	Expected Pleasure/ Satisfaction (0–100)	Actual Pleasure/ Satisfaction (0–100)	Comments
Example: Tuesday, 9:00 a.m.	yoga	40	60	Hard to get out of bed, but once I did it was better than expected.

As you try out activities, you may notice that you derive more pleasure or satisfaction from doing something than you originally predicted. If this is the case, keeping a record of what you do can reinforce doing that activity the next time that you are contemplating whether or not to engage in it, especially if you don't feel like it in the moment. Knowing that you usually feel much better afterward, even if it is the last thing you feel like doing in the moment, can serve as a great motivator. On the other hand, if you find you have tried an activity several times and do not get much pleasure or enjoyment from it, you can make the decision to try something else.

The Power of Exercise

Research has confirmed that exercise has multiple benefits that extend from enhancing your mood and fitness to reducing menopausal symptoms and improving your quality of life (Guimarães and Baptista 2011; Cardoso et al. 2011). Therefore, as you add new activities into your schedule, it's definitely worthwhile to consider a form of exercise. Of course, everyone is different in terms of activity level and restrictions, so if you are unsure about what level or type of exercise would be appropriate for you, you may want to discuss this with your doctor or a health care professional.

COGNITIVE STRATEGIES FOR CHANGING HOW YOU FEEL

You can also treat depression and other problematic feelings by tackling your thinking patterns. Some thoughts can be both problematic and distorted and can really contribute to how you feel in a negative way. Recall the connections within the CBT model:

Thought: *Things will never get any better.*

Feeling: depression

Behavior: withdrawal, avoidance

The thought in this example that *things will never get any better* is a common depressive thought that can elicit feelings of hopelessness and despair. It can also influence your behaviors or reactions, namely withdrawing from social or working activities. In other words, why would you do anything or put forth any energy if your thoughts are that nothing will get any better? To break this pattern, the first step is to recognize that your thought, in this case that *things will never get any better*, is distorted. This is a distorted thought simply because you cannot predict what the future holds; you are not a fortune-teller. Though at a certain point you may feel like nothing will get any better, it's inaccurate to make that definitive conclusion about the future.

Keeping a Thought Record

So how do you turn these thoughts around? You can start with keeping a thought record, where you identify your negative thoughts and look for cognitive distortions (see list in chapter 4). The following thought record shows how Catherine completed this exercise.

Catherine's Thought Record

Situation	Feelings (0–100)	Thoughts	Cognitive Distortions
Hearing about my coworker's daughter's wedding and recognizing that I will never experience this.	depressed (90) despair (70)	I made the wrong life choices and people must think I am crazy for choosing other things in life.	filtering catastrophizing personalizing fortune-telling

Over the course of the coming week, you can use the following thought record to examine your negative thoughts and look for negative distortions in your thinking. You may want to make photocopies of the blank worksheet before you begin.

Your Thought Record

Over the next week, use the following thought record three to five times to practice recording your thoughts and analyzing them for cognitive distortions. First list the situation you were in. Then record your feelings and rate their intensity on a scale of 0 to 100 (where 0 is the least intense and 100 is the most intense). Record your thoughts (what was going through your mind before and after) and list any cognitive distortions that you can identify in your thinking.

Situation	Feelings (0–100)	Thoughts	Cognitive Distortions

Changing Your Thoughts

Now that you have identified your thoughts and cognitive distortions, you can learn how to change your thoughts. It is not enough to change a thought from negative to positive. An example of this would be to take a thought like *I made the wrong life choices* and change it to *Everything is great!* or *This is the best day of my life!* Sure, these thoughts are positive, but they are as distorted as the negative thought. The fact is that everything is not great right now, and this is probably not the best day of your life either.

When distressed, you may experience automatic thoughts that, while they are partially true, are skewed and gear you in a negative direction. This is because you are not considering all the possibilities in that moment.

Examining the Evidence

A more effective way to change your thoughts from distorted and negative thoughts—thoughts that have a negative influence on how you feel and make it difficult to cope—is to come up with alternative ways of thinking about things. More specifically, you want to examine all of the evidence supporting your negative thoughts, as well as all the evidence against these negative thoughts, and then come up with alternative thoughts that reflect what you've learned. Taking the following steps can be helpful:

1. Identify a negative thought.

2. List all of the evidence you can find that either supports (evidence for) and/or disproves (evidence against) the negative thought.

3. Based on the evidence, conclude with an alternative, more balanced thought.

Catherine expanded her thought record to examine the evidence for and against some of her negative thoughts and to come up with alternative thoughts. The following example shows how she did this with one of these thoughts.

Catherine's Thought Record: Examining the Evidence

Situation	Feelings (0–100)	Thoughts	Evidence Supporting Negative Thought	Evidence against Negative Thought	Alternative Thoughts
In the staff room during the lunch hour on Wednesday, listening to my coworkers talk about a new grandchild and a daughter's upcoming wedding	depressed (90) despair (70)	I made the wrong life choices and people must think I am crazy for choosing other things in life.	I chose not to have children. Others have asked me why I made this choice. Others appear so happy with their children. Others appear balanced with work and children. Others have exciting life events, such as having grandchildren and attending weddings of their children.	Just because I made this choice does not make it wrong. When people ask me why I made this choice, it doesn't mean they think I am crazy. They could just be curious, as it is a decision that deviates from the norm. Until recently, I was happy and confident in my choice too. I never found the right partner I wanted to share that with and did not want to raise children on my own. I have also been very dedicated to the children I teach. I have been recognized with awards for teaching and make a difference guiding young children as a teacher. I enjoy a balance between work and family life.	Just because I chose not to have children, which might be a deviation from the norm, does not mean it is a wrong decision, nor does it make me crazy. Although it may seem to others that my life is not balanced, not everyone knows the details of my life and how involved I am with my family, especially my nieces and nephews. My work as a special needs teacher as of late is important and exciting to me. I have many other fulfilling activities in my life.

You can use the following worksheet to help you come up with alternative thoughts whenever your thoughts are distorted and negative. Before you begin, you may want to photocopy the blank worksheet for later use.

Your Thought Record: Examining the Evidence

Record the situation you were in, the feelings you had and their intensity on a 0 to 100 scale (where 0 is the least intense and 100 is the most intense), and your thoughts. Then focus on one of the negative thoughts you have identified and write down the evidence supporting it and the evidence against it. Based on the evidence, come up with more balanced alternatives.

Situation	Feelings (0–100)	Thoughts	Evidence Supporting Negative Thought	Evidence against Negative Thought	Alternative Thoughts

Dealing with Depression and Other Feelings

Moving Forward

What you need to do going forward with these strategies is practice, practice, and practice some more! Whenever you notice your mood going down, you can use the worksheets provided in this chapter to help you continue to track your thoughts, identity any cognitive distortions, and come up with alternative ways of thinking. With practice, you'll get better at countering your negative distorted thinking. The ultimate goal is for you to automatically take these cognitive steps as you encounter challenging moments.

SUMMING IT ALL UP

- The menopausal transition can be a time of heightened risk for women to develop depressive symptoms or clinical depression, either as a first onset or as a recurrent episode. Vasomotor symptoms and disrupted sleep can contribute to mood problems, but mood changes can also occur independently of these other symptoms.

- There are a number of effective treatments for depression and other menopause-related complaints, including antidepressants, estrogen therapy, and psychological treatments, such as CBT.

- Recognizing the stressors in your life, as well as the activities and thoughts that are contributing to your depression, might be a necessary step toward recovery.

- Specific CBT techniques, such as behavioral activation and use of thought records, are effective psychological components of therapy for depression.

CHAPTER 8

Getting a Good Night's Sleep

How common is sleep disruption during menopause?

What are some important variables to consider in the sleep environment?

How can changing my behaviors improve my sleep hygiene?

What other strategies could I use for hot flashes, night sweats, and anxiety?

This chapter will discuss common sleep-related problems associated with the menopausal transition and provide strategies to reduce the impact that sleep disruption has on your life. Understanding what's getting in the way of a good night's sleep is the first step toward solving the problem. This chapter starts off with some basic facts about sleep disruption and its consequences during menopause. Then it provides you with tools to monitor your sleep-related habits over time so that you can analyze your sleep patterns. Finally, it offers some tips on good sleep hygiene and some behavioral and cognitive strategies that you can use to get a better night's sleep.

SLEEP DISRUPTION

Sleeplessness, also known as *insomnia*, can include difficulties falling asleep and the inability to stay asleep through the night; one can experience poor sleep quality or quantity, or premature or constant awakenings without being able to resume sleep. These difficulties can last a few days or a few weeks, or insomnia can be chronic, occurring at least three nights a week for a month or longer.

The term *primary insomnia* refers to a sleep disorder that's not related to a medical, psychiatric, or environmental cause. *Secondary insomnia*, which is sleep disruption due to medical conditions, psychological factors such as anxiety, or medicines or substances, is more common and often resolves with treatment. Menopause-related sleep disruption would fall in this latter category.

Obesity, high blood pressure, age, use of caffeine and drugs or alcohol, inactivity, and a work schedule that disrupts your internal clock are all considered overall risk factors for disruption in sleep.

Oftentimes, people ask what is the appropriate amount of sleep that one should aim for during the night. Sleep is considered adequate if you can function in an alert state while awake. For most people, this means obtaining roughly six to nine hours of sleep each night (North American Menopause Society 2010b).

Sleep Disruption and Menopause

According to the National Sleep Foundation (NSF) survey, about 61 percent of menopausal women have sleep problems. The NSF survey also revealed that perimenopausal and postmenopausal women sleep less and have more frequent insomnia symptoms compared to premenopausal women (National Sleep Foundation 2010).

Night sweats can result in significant sleep disruption (Woodward and Freeman 1994). Women who awake in the night due to night sweats can find it difficult to get back to sleep. It is important to note, however, that women may experience disrupted sleep at this stage in life even in the absence of hot flashes at nighttime (Soares and Murray 2006).

Hormone fluctuations during menopause may also play a role in sleep disruption. More specifically, fluctuations in estrogen and progesterone may alter gamma-aminobutyric acid (GABA) function and play a role in menopause-related insomnia (Krystal 2004). GABA is a neurotransmitter that plays a central role in sleep initiation and maintenance.

Psychological factors during this time of life, including stress, anxiety, and depression, are linked to an inability to fall or stay asleep and may share common underlying mechanisms (Soares and Murray 2006).

Important to note is that sleep laboratory studies that investigated common causes of sleep disturbance in perimenopausal and postmenopausal women identified a significant number of women with sleep-disordered breathing, or obstructive sleep apnea syndrome, and restless leg syndrome (Freedman and Roehrs 2007). Sleep apnea is a disorder in which you have one or more pauses in breathing, lasting seconds to minutes, while you sleep. Oftentimes, you move from deep sleep to light sleep, which affects the overall quality of your sleep. Diminishing progesterone levels during menopause may be a cause of sleep apnea, as progesterone is a known respiratory stimulant and upper airway dilator. Increased body weight associated with menopause and aging may also increase the risk for sleep apnea (Young et al. 1993). Restless leg syndrome is a disorder in which there is an urge or need to move the legs to stop an unpleasant sensation, which can result in a decrease in the quality of your sleep. Both sleep apnea and restless leg syndrome impact sleep efficiency and daytime functioning.

When assessed objectively (for example, with the use of sleep studies), sleep problems are commonly associated with sleep apnea as well as periodic limb movement and arousals. Poor subjective sleep quality, on the other hand, is often associated with anxiety, depression, and the number of hot flashes in the first half of the night (Freedman and Roehrs 2007).

Available Treatments

Sleep medications, such as eszopiclone (Lunesta) and zolpidem (Ambien), have been shown to be helpful in menopause-associated insomnia (Soares et al. 2006; Dorsey, Lee, and Scharf 2004). These treatment options, however, are seen as temporary solutions.

CBT has been shown to be more effective than sleep medication in controlling some types of insomnia (Jacobs et al. 2004). By improving sleep habits and challenging counterproductive misconceptions about sleep, CBT may be a useful tool in tackling insomnia during the menopausal years.

> **Quick Check**
>
> If you find that you are getting enough sleep at night but continue to be sleepy throughout the day and suspect a sleep disorder, such as sleep apnea, restless leg syndrome, or narcolepsy (a nervous system disorder causing excessive sleepiness), speak with your family doctor. You may be referred to a sleep center for testing, diagnosis, and treatment.

HOW SLEEP DISRUPTION AFFECTS YOU

In the CBT model, presented in figure 8.1, poor sleep is a behavior that can interfere with your ability to cope with the day's activities as well as other menopausal symptoms.

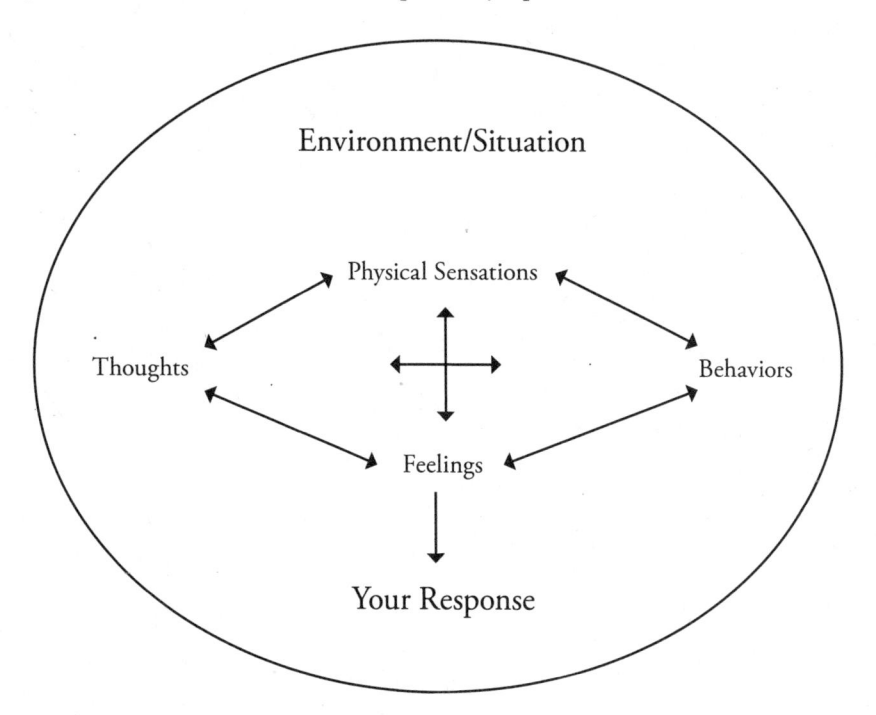

Figure 8.1: The CBT model

More specifically, poor sleep can result in not only an increase in fatigue but also difficulties with concentration and problematic mood states such as anxiety, irritability, and depression.

Behavior (poor sleep) ⟶ **Feelings** (irritability, anxiety)

Physical sensation (fatigue)

Thought (*This will never get any better.*)

This chapter will give you some cognitive and behavioral methods to improve your sleep patterns, but first you will need to look more closely at how you sleep.

Monitoring Your Sleep Patterns

Keeping a sleep diary can give you a better understanding of your sleep patterns (Carney and Manber 2009). Gloria's diary gives examples of the type of information that you will want to collect.

Gloria's Sleep Diary

	Monday	Tuesday	Wednesday	Thursday	Friday	Saturday	Sunday
What time did you go to bed? Were you tired?	11:00 p.m. Yes	12:00 a.m. Yes	10:00 p.m. No	10:00 p.m. No	12:30 a.m. Yes	11:00 p.m. Yes	11:30 p.m. Yes
How long did it take you to fall asleep? Did you leave the bedroom if it was more than fifteen minutes?	15 minutes	5 minutes	45 minutes No	1 hour No	5 minutes	15 minutes	10 minutes
If you woke during the night, how much time did you spend awake? What did you do?	30 minutes Stayed in bed	45 minutes Went to living room and watched "thriller" movie	30 minutes Stayed in bed	1 hour Went to living room and watched "Fear Factor"	30 minutes Stayed in bed	1 hour Answered e-mails and surfed web	1 hour Surfed the web
What time did you wake in the morning?	7:00 a.m.	8:00 a.m.	8:30 a.m.	7:45 a.m.	9:00 a.m.	8:00 a.m.	8:15 a.m.
What time did you actually get out of bed in the morning?	7:30 a.m.	8:15 a.m.	8:30 a.m.	8:00 a.m.	9:00 a.m.	8:30 a.m.	8:30 a.m.

Over the next two weeks, you can use the following sleep diary to monitor your sleep. Before you begin, you will need to make at least one photocopy.

Your Sleep Diary

Over the next week, keep track of your sleep patterns by answering the following questions after every night's sleep.

	Monday	Tuesday	Wednesday	Thursday	Friday	Saturday	Sunday
What time did you go to bed? Were you tired?							
How long did it take you to fall asleep? Did you leave the bedroom if it was more than fifteen minutes?							
If you woke during the night, how much time did you spend awake? What did you do?							
What time did you wake in the morning?							
What time did you actually get out of bed in the morning?							

Analyzing Your Sleep Diary

After completing your sleep diary for two weeks, you can probably recognize certain patterns as you look at the different entries. Here's what Gloria learned from this exercise.

Gloria's Sleep Diary Analysis

1. What time did you go to bed? Were you tired?

   There were a couple of nights that I did not go to bed when I was tired. I went to bed those nights anyway because my husband was retiring to bed and I felt like joining him.

2. How long did it take you to fall asleep? Did you leave the bedroom if it was more than fifteen minutes?

   It took me a substantial amount of time to fall asleep during the times I went to bed when I was not tired. Sometimes up to one hour. I always stayed in bed, though.

3. Did you wake up during the night? What did you do?

   I always seem to wake up in the night—anywhere from thirty minutes to an hour. Half the time, I stay in bed and find that my busy mind (whether it is planning for the next day or trying to resolve a problem) is consuming and prevents me from falling asleep again. If I get up, I engage in an activity that is stimulating or productive. At least I am getting something done while I am awake.

4. What time did you wake up in the morning? What time did you actually get out of bed?

   My wake time varies depending on how tired I am. My responsibilities differ every day too, and some days I do not have to be anywhere, so I will stay in bed.

Your Sleep Diary Analysis

Review the entries in your diary and look for any regular patterns. Then answer the following:

1. What time did you go to bed? Were you tired?

   _____
   _____
   _____

2. How long did it take you to fall asleep? Did you leave the bedroom if it was more than fifteen minutes?

   _____
   _____
   _____

3. Did you wake up during the night? What did you do?

   _____
   _____
   _____

4. What time did you wake up in the morning? What time did you actually get out of bed?

   _____
   _____
   _____

MAINTAINING GOOD SLEEP HYGIENE

Sleep hygiene refers to the act of controlling all behavioral and environmental factors that may influence the length and quality of your sleep. Understanding and practicing good sleep hygiene is essential to ensure a restorative night's sleep. This section will cover some factors that may be affecting your sleep patterns and help you examine whether your sleep habits are consistent with good sleep hygiene. If not, you can make some changes that may improve your sleep.

Your Sleep Environment

Modifying your environment may help you get a better night's sleep. Several variables may be having an effect on your sleep. If you look over the following list of possibilities and think about your own sleep environment, you can probably determine what kinds of changes might improve your sleep.

Temperature: What is the temperature of the room you sleep in? Is it particularly warm? Do you find yourself throwing your covers off in the middle of the night? If so, you may want to adjust the thermostat in your house before you go to bed, so you are sleeping at a comfortable temperature. Regardless of whether it is the middle of summer or the coldest month of the year, finding a temperature that is not disruptive can be very helpful both for the quality of sleep you get and in preventing you from waking up and having to adjust.

Light source: Are you sleeping in a dark room, or do you find that there is light streaming through your bedroom window or doorway? Arranging your bedroom so that any source of light is extinguished and your room remains dark can be helpful. The traditional culprits include nightlights, bathroom lights, and hallway lights, which can illuminate the room to a point that is disruptive. Furthermore, it is important to consider street lights and even the moon at certain times of the year, as these can be a light source that impacts your sleep environment.

Noises: Is it your tendency to start the dishwasher right before going to bed? Perhaps you have an old grandfather clock that chimes on the half hour, or you hear the bus drive by your open window. Noises, however minimal, can contribute to problems with sleep by keeping you up or waking you up several times during the night. In order to minimize the chance of staying awake or waking up, make sure that your sleep environment is quiet by turning off appliances, such as the washer/dryer and dishwasher, adjusting clocks, and keeping the TV and radio off in the bedroom.

Sleeping surface: How old is your mattress? Is your pillow comfortable? Is your bedding too soft, too hard, or just right? Goldilocks had it right in continuing her search for the perfect bed prior to curling up in hopes of a good sleep. These are important questions to consider. A mattress that is too old, too stiff, or too soft can affect your quality of sleep, as can a pillow that gives you a headache rather than comfort and layers of bedding that get to be too much.

> ## Quick Check
>
> What are a couple of modifications that you can make in your sleep environment that might make it more comfortable and make getting a good night's sleep easier?
>
> 1.
>
> 2.

Bedtime-Related Activities

Though sleep disruptions can start out as the result of menopause or menopause-related symptoms such as night sweats, behavioral habits can often contribute significantly to perpetuating the problem. Behavioral modifications that are consistent with good sleep hygiene can help remedy some of the disruptions you may be experiencing with sleep (Harvey 2000).

Eliminate daytime naps: On the surface it seems to make sense that if you are tired during the day, you should take a nap, especially if you are having difficulties with sleep at night. This behavior can actually sabotage your efforts to get a good sleep come nighttime. When you take a nap during the day, it offsets the rhythm and routine that you are striving toward with your body. For instance, having a nap during the day can result in being less tired at night when you would normally go to bed. This can, in turn, affect how quickly you fall asleep and when you wake up (either being too tired to wake up when you want to or sleeping in longer than you intended). It's better to fight through the fatigue during the day and go to bed at an appropriate time at night.

Establish a bedtime routine: When you establish a ritual before going to bed, your body begins to learn the different cues that it is time to wind down and relax. For instance, maybe you make your lunch for the next day in the quiet kitchen and empty the dishwasher before heading to the washroom to change into your bedtime wear and brush your teeth. If you establish a bedtime routine, whatever it is, over time your body will associate these activities with preparing for sleep, which can certainly facilitate sleep.

Go to bed when you are tired: If you find that you tend to go to bed at a certain time every night, even if you are not too tired, you may want to reconsider this. By going to bed when you notice the signs of sleepiness and fatigue from your body (for example, heavy eyelids, yawning, difficulty keeping your head up), as opposed to letting the clock dictate when you head to bed, the likelihood of falling asleep is greater. On the other hand, if you go to bed when you do not feel tired, you risk staying awake in bed longer. This can lead to negative associations between your bed and unsuccessful efforts to fall asleep.

The fifteen-minute rule: If you find that you are awake in bed for longer than fifteen minutes from the time you attempted to fall asleep, get up! Your body very quickly starts to make an association between being awake and being in bed, which interferes with your efforts to fall asleep when you head to bed. In order to try to prevent this from happening, get out of bed after about fifteen minutes. Remove yourself from the bedroom and engage in a quiet, nonstimulating activity until you start to feel sleepy again.

Avoid stimulating and strenuous activities before bedtime: Engaging in stimulating or strenuous activities close to bedtime is a bad idea. Doing something physical, like exercise, or cognitively stimulating, like talking on the phone or watching an action movie, close to a desired sleep time has the potential to increase arousal and make it difficult for you to fall asleep. It's important to get regular exercise, as well as a good dose of stimulating activities during the day. However, if you have been engaging in these types of activities close to bedtime, you may want to adjust your schedule to ensure that they are not interfering with your sleep.

Reserve the bedroom for sleep and intimacy: Do you eat the occasional meal in bed, read or watch TV tucked under the covers, or just hang out on your bed talking on the phone? All of these activities have the potential for your body and mind to associate being awake and being in bed. It is important to use your bed only for of sleeping or intimacy so that you can minimize unwanted wakeful times at night.

Refrain from eating or drinking prior to going to bed: If you find that you frequently wake to use the bathroom at night, you may wish to restrict the amount of fluids that you drink before bed. For instance, if you tend to head to bed at about 10:00 p.m., you may want to stop drinking fluids by 8:00 p.m. Furthermore, eating something before bed will mean that your digestive system is now busy doing its job.

Beware of caffeine, alcohol, and nicotine intake: Being mindful of what you consume a few hours prior to going to bed can make a difference in how well you sleep. For instance, drinking caffeinated beverages or eating anything that might have caffeine in it a few hours before bed can prevent you from falling asleep. It takes about fifteen to thirty minutes for caffeine from a cup of coffee to affect the brain, and up to seven hours are required for your system to eliminate the caffeine; its stimulant effects may last for up to twenty hours (Landolt et al. 1995). Besides being found in coffee, caffeine is often present in tea, energy drinks, cola drinks, and chocolate. It is also present in some nonprescription medications, such as pain relievers, allergy medications, and cold medications. As such, bringing more attention to what you consume in the afternoon and evening before going to bed has the potential to reduce the impact of sleep disruption. With respect to alcohol, although it initially may make you feel a little on the drowsy side and can assist with falling asleep, it often results in rebound early awakening and fragmented sleep, leading to feeling not refreshed upon awakening. Alcohol also affects breathing and tends to swell oral and nasal mucous membranes. Nicotine has been observed to prolong sleep onset and decrease sleep duration.

Get up at the same time every day: Even when you stayed up late the night before and can, in theory, afford to sleep in, it is still imperative to wake up at the same time the next day! In order to ensure that you become tired at roughly the same time every night and wake up at the same time the next morning, you need to follow a schedule.

Specific Menopausal Behavioral Tips

In addition to practicing good sleep hygiene, taking the following actions will help you deal with vasomotor symptoms.

1. Wear lighter pajamas to bed.

2. Keep a second pair of pajamas near the bed.

3. Minimize the bedding that you have or use lighter bedding.

4. Keep a fan nearby.

5. Keep a cool beverage near the bed.

Doing these things should help you sleep better if you suffer from night sweats. More generally, you may want to analyze your sleep diary once more to see if you can make other improvements to your sleep environment or before-bedtime activity.

What You Can Do Differently

After reviewing your sleep diary once more, what adjustments could you make to try to improve your sleep? Write down the possibilities.

1. _____

2. _____

3. _____

4. _____

MAKING BEHAVIORAL CHANGES

Based on what you've learned in this chapter, you may be ready to make some changes to improve your sleep hygiene. You may have the urge to make a lot of changes at once, but it will be better to start with one or two. This way you will avoid feeling overwhelmed. Plus, it will be easier to decide whether the strategies you've chosen are helpful or not if you are tweaking only a couple things at a time.

The best way to evaluate the results is to treat making changes as an experiment in which you decide on a strategy, implement it, and record the results. You should try any new strategy for roughly a week to determine whether it has been helpful or not. Based on the results, you can choose to keep the change or discard it. In either case, once you've evaluated the effectiveness of the changes you've made, you can try making other changes as well.

You can use the following worksheet to record the results of your experiments with behavior modification. Before you begin, you may want to photocopy the blank worksheet for later use.

Behavior Modification Experiment

Record the dates that you are trying out a new behavior or technique, the behavior or technique you've chosen to try, and the outcome (if you noticed any change or if you found the new behavior or technique helpful). Give the new strategy about a week to determine its effectiveness.

Date	Behavior/Technique Chosen	Outcome

Once you've tried out one or two new behaviors and recorded the results over a period of time, you should know whether you want to continue to implement them. You can continue to experiment in this way with other new behaviors to see if they improve your sleep patterns.

PSYCHOLOGICAL FACTORS AND SLEEP DISRUPTION

While certain behaviors can have a negative impact on your ability to fall asleep and stay asleep, your thoughts and reactions to stress and anxiety can also prove problematic. Sleep researchers found that people with insomnia have more anxious thoughts and negative emotions than good sleepers do (Harvey and Farrell 2003). If you find that you are up experiencing worry thoughts and trying to resolve problems in your mind at 3:00 a.m., here are some strategies to reduce your worries and associated arousal.

Get out of bed and leave the bedroom: If you are not sleeping within about fifteen minutes (in this case due to an overactive mind), then get out of bed and leave the bedroom. Even further, if you realize that your mind is overactive to begin with, then it is not necessary to wait a full fifteen minutes before getting out of bed. Again, pairing an arousing activity, such as thinking, with being in bed will encourage your brain to associate the two. Return to bed only when you feel tired again.

Keep a pen and paper on the nightstand: Worrying at 3:00 a.m. about the things you have to do the next day not only interferes in the sleep process but is pointless, since you can't do anything about these things that you're thinking about. For instance, you may decide that you need to contact the cable company to change your subscription, but unfortunately no one is going to be there at 3:00 a.m. to answer your call. You may find it helpful to spend some time every night before bed writing about your thoughts and concerns. Harvey and Farrell (2003) found that those who engaged in such journaling fell asleep more quickly compared to those who did not. You may also want to leave your pen and paper (or journal) on your nightstand in the event that you begin to worry about something during the night. This way, you can tell yourself that once you wake up, you will tend to this issue and thus lay to rest your fear that you'll forget.

Schedule worry time in the day: Try solving problems during the day when you are more likely to be effective. Researchers have found that scheduling worry time into your day can reduce mental overactivity at night in people with poor sleep (Carney and Waters 2006). For instance, you might want to reserve a half hour each morning or an hour in the afternoon to focus on your concerns and on potential solutions. This strategy would work well coupled with the previous strategy of keeping a pen and paper on the nightstand, since you can use the pen and paper at night to jot down reminders of what to think about the next day.

Focus on the breath: As a form of redirection and relaxation, it can be helpful to focus on the breath. Your mind might jump back to a worry thought a hundred times, but bringing it back to the breath just as many times can be useful as a means of cognitive distraction (Waters et al. 2003).

Listen to relaxation CDs: If you have found that a relaxation CD has been helpful in the past, you may want to reintroduce it here. Relaxation CDs that have formal practices on them, such as progressive muscle relaxation, guided imagery, and diaphragmatic breathing, have been shown to be very effective as part of a treatment protocol for clinical anxiety disorders. Therefore using them might be helpful as a means of winding down before bed.

COGNITIVE STRATEGIES FOR A BETTER NIGHT'S SLEEP

Recall the thought-behavior-feeling connection from the CBT model. Specific thoughts that you have about sleep can influence how you feel and ultimately how much (or little) sleep you get. For example, the thought *I won't be able to function if I don't go to sleep now* can lead to a feeling of anxiety, a physical sensation of tension, and a behavior of tossing and turning.

In fact, the thought *I won't be able to function if I don't go to sleep now* represents one of several common cognitive distortions about sleep that can perpetuate your inability to get to sleep and increase your distress. If you can recognize such cognitive distortions in your own thoughts, you can counter them with some alternative thoughts that will make sleeping easier.

The following are some common sleep-interfering categories of cognitive distortions:

Failure to function: Such thoughts as *I won't be able to function if I don't go to sleep now* and *I will be useless tomorrow if I don't get a good night's sleep* fall within this category. Research has shown that compared to people without sleep problems, people with insomnia perform just as well on basic mental tasks (Bonnet 2005). So, although they find it more challenging, people with insomnia can manage to mentally get through the day.

Misplaced effort: Included in this category are such thoughts as *I have to do something to make sure I get to sleep*. You may experience a great deal of anxiety over getting less than a specific amount of sleep per night, as you believe that there is a certain type of mental effort required to get to sleep. What is more helpful is understanding that the body knows what it needs and relying on it to take care of itself!

Intolerability: The general belief in this category is that lost sleep or difficulties falling asleep will be a horrible experience. Such thoughts as *I cannot stand this* and *this will be unbearable tonight* are common and negatively affect how the night will unfold. In fact, you might not have even gone to bed and yet are preparing for the worst. Such negative thinking can turn out to be a self-fulfilling prophecy, which can make trying to fall asleep more difficult. However, although difficult, your struggle to fall asleep is an experience that you've gotten through before and will get through again.

Unnecessary desire: In this category, thoughts like *I really want eight hours of sleep* may cause anxiety. Sleep want is not the same as sleep need. In reality, there is no magic number of hours we all need to engage in to ensure proper rest and function the next day. Rather, the necessary amount of sleep varies from person to person.

Do you find yourself engaging in any of these cognitive distortions? A trend you might detect in these thoughts is a belief that you are unable to cope with less sleep or insomnia. An interesting fact is that people who have insomnia actually cope quite well in spite of their lack of sleep (Bonnet 2005).

Keeping a Thought Record

You can use a thought record to uncover some of the distressing thoughts or images that may be contributing to your sleep problems and to develop alternative thoughts. Keeping a thought record can help you develop alternative thoughts to use when distressing thoughts get in the way of sleep. Perhaps the best way to do this is to record the thoughts that were occupying your mind the night before as soon as you can the next day. The following thought record shows how Gloria did this exercise.

Gloria's Thought Record with Alternative Thoughts

Situation	Feelings (0–100)	Thoughts/Predictions	Cognitive Distortion	Alternative Thoughts
Woke up in night and couldn't fall back asleep	*anxious (70)*	*If I don't fall asleep now, I will not be able to get everything I need to get done tomorrow.* *I can't stand this. I should get up and get a few things done now since I can't sleep.*	*failure to function* *intolerability*	*It is more difficult to function the next day after a poor night's sleep, but I have always been able to get the most important tasks of the day done.*

Your Thought Record with Alternative Thoughts

Record a distressing situation that was related to sleep, the feelings you had at the time, and their intensity on a scale of 0 to 100 (where 0 is the least intense and 100 is the most intense). Write down what you thought at the time and any cognitive distortions in which you were engaging. Finally, using what you've learned in this chapter, come up with some more reasonable alternative thoughts that you might use when you are having difficulty sleeping.

Situation	Feelings (0–100)	Thoughts/Predictions	Cognitive Distortion	Alternative Thoughts

Ultimately, you want to use such alternative thoughts in place of cognitive distortions when you experience similar circumstances in the future. With time, these alternative thoughts will help reduce the distress you are experiencing and help you sleep.

MOVING FORWARD

Continuing to implement good sleep hygiene techniques, as well as implementing the behavioral and cognitive strategies proposed in this chapter that may be applicable to you, will help ensure, with time, better sleep. When keeping a thought record, remember to record the thoughts that were occupying your mind the night before as soon as you can the following day. With enough practice keeping a thought record, you will develop the ability to take these cognitive steps when you experience distress while trying to get to sleep!

SUMMING IT ALL UP

- According to the National Sleep Foundation, about 61 percent of menopausal women have sleep problems. Night sweats can result in significant sleep disruption (Woodward and Freeman 1994). However, other factors, including decline in estrogen and progesterone and stress, anxiety, and depression, are linked to an inability to fall asleep.

- Sleep disruption results in not only an increase in fatigue but difficulties with concentration and problematic mood states, such as anxiety, irritability, and depression. These, in turn, can interfere with your ability to cope with other menopausal symptoms.

- Cognitive behavioral therapy has been shown to be more effective than sleep medication in controlling insomnia (Jacobs et al. 2004).

- Good sleep hygiene strategies, including modifications to the sleep environment and before-bedtime routines, help ensure a good night's sleep.

- Behavioral modification strategies that are specific to menopause, anxiety, and stress can also reduce disruption in sleep.

- Reducing anxious arousal by addressing worries in the day and taking pressure off yourself to fall asleep can help promote a good night's rest.

CHAPTER 9

Addressing Urogenital Problems and Sexual Concerns

What are the common urogenital problems during menopause?

What are the common sexual concerns during menopause?

What are some effective behavioral strategies I can use?

What are some effective cognitive strategies I can use?

Urogenital problems and sexual concerns are common during the menopausal transition. You may have either of these concerns or both. The term *urogenital* refers to the involvement of both the urinary and genital structures and functions. Sexual concerns may include a decreased libido, or sex drive, or low motivation for sexual activity for a variety of reasons. During the menopausal transition, women may experience a number of urogenital problems and sexual concerns, and the information in this chapter is by no means exhaustive. The intent, rather, is to cover some of the more common urogenital problems and sexual concerns that you may be experiencing.

Again, it's important to understand the nature of any problem before attempting to solve or treat it. Perhaps reading about what women frequently report may help clarify what you are going through, or you may already have a good sense of what's troubling you. In either case, it is best to make an appointment with your family physician or health care provider to obtain confirmation and to use this workbook as a complementary method of treatment.

COMMON UROGENITAL PROBLEMS

Two of the most common urogenital problems that women experience during menopause are painful urination, also referred to as *dysuria,* and instances of involuntary loss of urine known as *urinary incontinence* (Hunskaar et al. 2000).

Vaginitis and vaginal atrophy are also common urogenital problems that occur during menopause. *Vaginitis* is the inflammation of vaginal tissues, while *vaginal atrophy* is when the lining of the vagina becomes thinner, drier, and less elastic or flexible (Mehta and Bachmann 2008). Both conditions may cause you to experience any of the following: vaginal dryness, itching, irritation, soreness, and pain during intercourse.

Causes of Urogenital Complaints

You may suffer from one or more urogenital complaints, each of which is caused by something different.

PAINFUL URINATION

Often the causes of painful urination during menopause are urinary tract infections. These include recurrent bladder infections, bladder inflammation and irritation, and bacterial infection of the urinary tract. A prolapsed bladder, which occurs when the bladder drops down into or outside of the vagina, can also be responsible for painful urination. Recurrent urinary tract infections during menopause can be due to a decrease in estrogen, which causes the bladder to become less elastic and can reduce its ability to fully empty. When urine is left in the bladder, the possibility for bacterial infection increases. Lower acidity levels in the bladder are also responsible for the increase in growth of bacteria resulting in urinary tract infections.

URINARY INCONTINENCE

The main risk factors for developing urinary incontinence include a depletion of estrogen, vaginal childbirth, and aging (Lukacz et al. 2011). During normal urination, the walls of the bladder contract and force urine from the bladder into the urethra (the short tube that passes urine from the bladder out of the body). The sphincter muscles surrounding the urethra relax, and the urine is allowed to pass and be excreted from the body. However, during the menopausal transition, a loss of estrogen can lead to thinning of the lining of the urethra (Hillard 2010). The surrounding pelvic muscles also weaken with aging and vaginal childbirth, a process known as pelvic relaxation. The most common types of urinary incontinence in women are stress incontinence and urge incontinence.

Stress incontinence involves the involuntary loss of small amounts of urine while laughing, sneezing, coughing, lifting objects, or exercising, caused by weakened pelvic floor muscles, which support the bladder and urethra. Although common during menopause, stress incontinence does not tend to worsen because of it. *Urge incontinence*, also known as *overactive bladder,* can be caused by an overly active bladder or irritated bladder muscles but can also be the result of damage to the nerves of the bladder. The most common symptom is involuntary loss of urine immediately after feeling the sudden urge to urinate. This may occur during sleep, after drinking a small amount of liquid, and when touching or hearing running water, such as when you do the dishes or hear a shower running.

VAGINITIS AND VAGINAL ATROPHY

Vaginitis and vaginal atrophy are associated with loss of estrogen (Robinson and Cardozo 2011). With regular levels of estrogen, vaginal secretions provide sufficient lubrication to prevent inflammation and atrophy. However, with reduced levels of estrogen comes a drop in vaginal secretions and decreased lubrication. Further, the possibility of the vagina becoming shorter and narrower increases when a woman does not have intercourse or other vaginal sexual activity on a regular basis following menopause. Infrequent intercourse is likely to be painful, since the dry, fragile vaginal tissues are susceptible to tearing and bleeding during intercourse.

> **Quick Check**
>
> Vaginal discomfort or painful urination can arise from many different sources. Check with your health care provider to determine the cause of persistent symptoms of dryness, irritation, burning, itchiness, or pain.

Treatment Options for Urogenital Complaints

For painful urination during menopause as a result of urinary tract infections, you can try modifying your diet, as well as make some behavioral changes in your urination habits that will be discussed later in this chapter. Painkillers might alleviate the discomfort, but the most important step is to properly treat the infection. Patients usually notice symptom relief within thirty-six hours of beginning treatment with antibiotics. Choosing the right antibiotic for each case depends on many factors: efficacy, risks of experiencing adverse effects, and treatment resistance (Colgan and Williams 2011).

For urinary incontinence, an ideal approach often requires the use of multiple treatment modalities, including behavioral therapy and lifestyle modifications, pelvic floor exercises, medications that should be discussed with your doctor, and surgical procedures including sling procedures that help keep the urethra closed (Gomelsky and Dmochowski 2011). Behavioral exercises that can help, including bladder drills and Kegel exercises, will be discussed later in this chapter.

For vaginitis and vaginal atrophy, continuing to have regular vaginal sexual activity throughout menopause and beyond can help keep vaginal tissues thick and moist and maintain the vagina's length and width (Sturdee and Panay 2010). Sexual stimulation can be helpful to increase vaginal secretions, and use of lubricants and moisturizers can decrease the friction on weakened vaginal structures (Palacios 2009). Finally, medications, such as a low dose of estrogen therapy in women who have no medical contraindications to its use, can restore vaginal blood flow, decrease acidity, and improve the thickness and elasticity of vaginal tissues (North American Menopause Society 2007).

COMMON SEXUAL CONCERNS

The World Health Organization (2012) defines sexual health as "a state of physical, emotional, mental, and social well-being in relation to sexuality; it is not merely the absence of disease, dysfunction, or infirmity." This definition recognizes that normal sexual response and function is different for everyone. Your sexual response and function is influenced socially by your culture, psychologically by your personal experiences, and physically by your biological makeup.

Although sexual health is very individualized, there are a few basic principles that contribute to a healthy sexual response and function for most people. These include an intact desire for sex, the ability to enjoy sex, and a comfort level with what and whom you sexually desire.

Your sexuality during the menopausal transition can be affected by a variety of factors, including biological changes, such as fluctuating hormone levels, and psychological and social factors. Although sexual problems generally increase with age, distressing sexual problems tend to peak in women aged forty-five to sixty-four (Lindau et al. 2007). Common sexual concerns reported by women during this time include the following:

- decreased sexual desire, also known as decreased libido
- decreased ability to become sexually aroused
- vaginal dryness or thinning of vaginal walls, causing pain during intercourse
- reduced ability to have an orgasm
- poor self-image and decreased sense of sexual attractiveness
- increased frequency of urinary tract infections

If you experience any of the above symptoms, there is potential for your sexual concerns to escalate. For instance, if you suffer from pain due to vaginitis, you may feel less attractive sexually and start to avoid sexual intimacy with your partner. This avoidance can result from fearing both pain during sexual activity and the sense of being less sexually desirable. This avoidance can lower your level of sexual desire and arousal.

Quick Check

Some sexual problems have a medical cause or may signal underlying medical conditions, such as urinary tract infections or dysuria. Speak to your health care provider regarding your sexual concerns, regardless of whether you consider them to be medical or not, to help determine the cause and appropriate treatment.

Common Contributors

Endless factors can contribute to decreased desire or motivation to engage in sexual activities. A few of the more common ones are listed below:

Urogenital problems: Vaginal discomfort or pain in the vulvovaginal structures, as well as urinary incontinence or urinary tract infections, can be a big contributor.

Hot flashes/night sweats: Severe hot flashes, even in the absence of psychological problems (symptoms of depression, anxiety), can be negatively associated with sexual activity (Nappi et al. 2010). The increase in body temperature that sexual activity can produce can either lead to a hot flash or have a negative impact on your desire to follow through with sexual intimacy.

Medical problems or side effects: Illness during the menopausal transition, including physical conditions and poor mental health, such as depression, can affect your overall well-being and interfere with sexual functioning. Further, some medications, including antidepressants, can have negative side effects on sexual desire and motivation.

Sleep disruption: Disruption in quantity or quality of sleep can leave you feeling tired, exhausted, or irritable and eventually result in less energy and desire to engage in sex.

Poor self-image and bodily changes: Both aging and depletion of estrogen can impact your appearance and ultimately your self-image. With age, your metabolism begins to slow, resulting in changes in weight and fat distribution and loss of muscle tone, including pelvic relaxation. Skin and hair changes occur with the depletion of estrogen and imbalance of other hormones.

Treatment Options for Sexual Concerns

You should speak with your family physician or health care provider when vaginitis, vaginal atrophy, dysuria, or urinary incontinence is present. These physical problems can not only contribute to sexual concerns but also compromise your physical health if left untreated. This chapter will discuss some behavioral strategies that can complement other treatment for these physical conditions.

This chapter will also discuss a number of behavioral modifications and cognitive strategies to help with sexual concerns that may or may not be influenced by urogenital problems. For example, changing your diet and getting more exercise can be effective for targeting both self-image and physical changes that occur. Furthermore, addressing beliefs that you have about yourself and your sexuality through cognitive strategies can have a large impact on your desire and motivation to engage in sexual activities.

As you can see within the CBT model, presented in figure 9.1, physical sensations that result from urogenital difficulties can affect how you feel, what you do, and how you think.

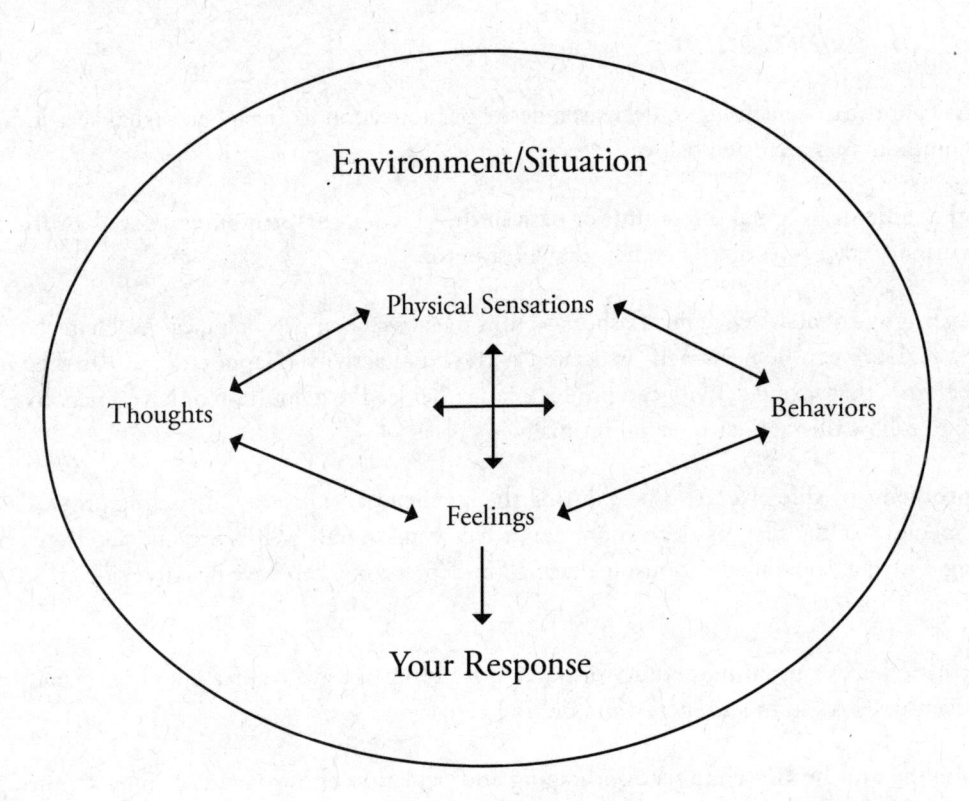

The Cognitive Behavioral Workbook for Menopause

Figure 9.1: The CBT model

Now that you have gained more of an understanding of the urogenital problems and sexual concerns that commonly occur during the menopausal transition, it will be helpful to reflect on what might be contributing to your difficulties. Becoming more aware of the links between your physical sensations or symptoms and your thoughts, feelings, and behaviors associated with them can be very helpful. For example, Ellen began to notice that she was having pain and tears from vaginal atrophy. As she wrote in her diary about it, she saw that these symptoms were influencing her thoughts, feelings, and behaviors.

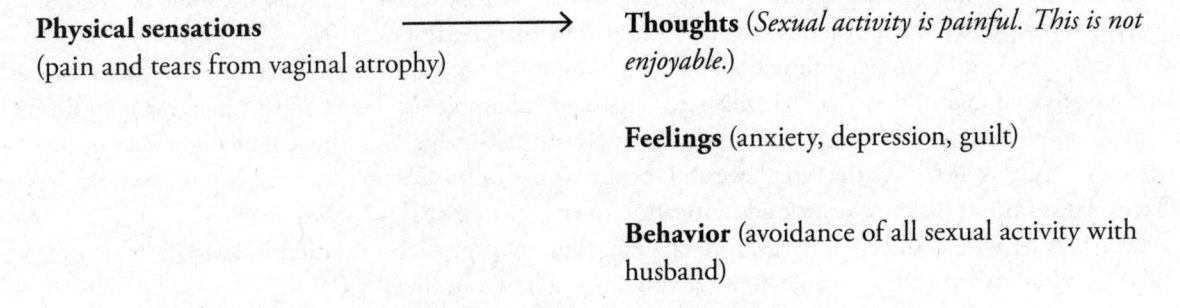

Physical sensations ⟶ **Thoughts** (*Sexual activity is painful. This is not enjoyable.*)
(pain and tears from vaginal atrophy)

Feelings (anxiety, depression, guilt)

Behavior (avoidance of all sexual activity with husband)

INCREASING YOUR AWARENESS

Increasing your awareness of the problem can help you figure out what to do about it. The next exercise will help you examine how urogenital problems or sexual concerns may be affecting your life. Here's how Ellen completed this exercise.

Ellen's Awareness Diary

1. What types of physical discomforts or sensations are you experiencing? What are the sexual concerns that you are having?

   Aside from the early postpartum years when I was heavily involved in the care of my babies and noticed a short-term drop in my libido, I have never experienced a problem with my sexuality or sexual intercourse. My husband and I have always had an enjoyable sexual relationship. Over the past six months, though, sexual intercourse has become quite painful for me. I started noticing that I am drier than usual when my husband and I engage in sex, and there have even been a couple times that tearing has occurred while having intercourse.

2. How are these concerns affecting you sexually? How are they affecting the rest of your life, including any romantic relationship you may have?

   When I first started noticing this problem, I just tried to ignore it, but after a while, it got so painful that I could not hide my discomfort. I started to become fearful over the next time I got intimate with my husband, knowing it would be painful and upsetting. It has gotten so bad now that my husband and I have not had sex in the last three months, and any time that he tries to engage in some sort of sexual intimacy, I withdraw immediately, fearing that it will lead to intercourse and, ultimately, pain. So for the past three months, my husband and I have not been close physically. We don't even hug anymore, and we certainly don't talk about it.

3. What are your thoughts and beliefs about this problem and the effect it has had on your life?

   The lack of sexual intimacy has really had a negative impact on my relationship with my husband. Having a strong sexual relationship was a way that we could both show how much we loved and cared for each other. Since this has not been happening, I fear that he does not love or care about me as much. We are not communicating as much as we used to, which makes me fear that the relationship is in jeopardy. I also do not believe I am as sexually appealing or attractive as I used to be and worry that this pain will never go away.

4. What are you doing to treat these concerns at this time?

   After speaking with a close friend of mine who disclosed that she had a similar experience, I made an appointment with my family doctor so that she can formally diagnose my physical problem and perhaps recommend some treatment options for the pain. I have also decided to initiate a conversation with my husband about this so that we can let each other know how we are feeling.

Clearly, Ellen is suffering from vaginal atrophy, and this urogenital problem led to significant sexual concerns and stopping any sexual intimacy with her husband. This interaction of a urogenital problem and sexual concerns is common, one often leading to the other. Only upon reflection did Ellen recognize these links and start to develop a plan of action that began with seeing her family physician for confirmation of diagnosis and a treatment plan.

Addressing Urogenital Problems and Sexual Concerns

Your Awareness Diary

Answer the following questions to increase your awareness of your urogenital problems or sexual concerns.

1. What types of physical discomforts or sensations are you experiencing? What are the sexual concerns that you are having?

   _____
   _____
   _____
   _____

2. How are these concerns affecting you sexually? How are they affecting the rest of your life, including any romantic relationship you may have?

   _____
   _____
   _____
   _____

3. What are your thoughts and beliefs about this problem and the effect it has had on your life?

   _____
   _____
   _____
   _____

4. What are you doing to treat these concerns at this time?

   _____
   _____
   _____
   _____

The rest of this chapter focuses on CBT strategies to help you cope better with the urogenital complaints or sexual concerns that you have.

BEHAVIORAL STRATEGIES FOR COPING WITH UROGENITAL COMPLAINTS

If you have been diagnosed with a urinary tract infection, dysuria, vaginitis, or vaginal atrophy, you may want to consider some behavioral strategies to complement other treatment that you may be receiving. Whichever of the following strategies you decide to engage in, we encourage you to discuss the strategy with your doctor and track your use of this strategy to evaluate its impact.

Preventing Urinary Tract Infections

Painful urination, in most cases, is a result of urinary tract infections. To avoid these, you may consider trying the following methods.

IMPROVED URINATION HABITS

When urine stays in the bladder too long, bacteria has the potential to grow, which increases the risk for a urinary tract infection. Therefore, urinating frequently and whenever the urge arises can be used as a preventative technique. You should also urinate shortly after having sex in order to flush away bacteria that could have entered into the urethra during intercourse. Wiping habits are also important to consider. After urinating, it is best to wipe from front to back to prevent bacteria from entering into the urethra.

FLUIDS AND NUTRITION

Drinking a lot of fluids, water in particular, can help flush bacteria from your system. The exact amounts should be discussed with your health care provider. Other fluids that have been found to be helpful as a proactive or preventative measure are cranberry juice and lingonberry juice.

LOOSE CLOTHING

It may help to wear loose-fitting clothing, or clothing that will allow airflow to keep the area around the urethra dry. Tighter-fitting clothes have the potential to trap moisture and help bacteria grow, which increases the risk of a urinary tract infection.

Vaginitis and Vaginal Atrophy

The following measures may prevent or help with vaginitis and vaginal atrophy.

REGULAR VAGINAL SEXUAL ACTIVITY

This includes sexual activity with or without penetration on a regular basis throughout menopause. This strategy can be helpful in keeping the vaginal tissues thick and moist. Regular penetrative sexual activity can also maintain the vagina's length and width.

MAXIMIZING STIMULATION

This can be done through use of self or mutual masturbation. Use of a vibrator to maximize stimulation can also be helpful to increase vaginal secretions.

NONHORMONAL THERAPY

Use of vaginal lubricants and moisturizers can decrease the friction on weakened vaginal structures that often leads to painful tearing.

Urinary Incontinence

You can try the following methods to help with the problem of urinary incontinence. Some exercises follow.

WEARING PADS OR PROTECTIVE GARMENTS

This strategy can be considered as more of a short-term solution. It can be helpful in maintaining freedom in activities that you choose to engage in and reducing worry over whether incontinence will occur.

KEGEL EXERCISES

For stress incontinence, the use of physical therapy in the form of Kegel exercises can make a substantial difference. The goal of Kegel exercises is to increase the strength of the pelvic floor muscles. These exercises involve contracting and relaxing the muscles of your pelvic floor: the area that holds your uterus and bladder in place above your vagina.

How to Do Kegel Exercises

1. While you are urinating, stop the flow of urine midstream. (Note: you should not do this on a regular basis, as stopping the flow of urine too often may actually worsen urinary incontinence. The point is to isolate the muscles that you will want to exercise later, when not urinating.)

2. Once you are able to isolate these muscles, contract them—without contracting any of the surrounding muscles in the abdomen or thighs—and hold the contraction for three seconds, release for three seconds, and repeat ten times.

3. Eventually, you will be able to contract and release the muscles for five-second intervals, which is a good goal. Whenever you practice, repeat ten times.

4. Practice three to four times per day or as often as possible. The more you engage in this exercise, the stronger these muscles will become.

In addition to strengthening pelvic floor muscles, Kegel exercises have resulted in other benefits, including awareness of the muscles involved in pleasurable sexual sensations, reduction of vaginal or pelvic pain during sex, improving urinary continence, and preventing/treating pelvic organ prolapse (Bo et al. 1990).

BLADDER DRILLS

For urge incontinence, engaging in bladder drills (timed voiding) can be helpful for retraining the bladder and ultimately reducing incontinence. The purpose is to increase the length of time between urinations, increase the amount of urine your bladder can hold, and diminish the sense of urgency or leakage that you experience.

How to Do Bladder Drills

Take the following steps over a twelve-day period.

1. Days 1–3: After awakening, empty your bladder every hour on the hour, even if you do not feel the need to go. Be sure to drink fluids frequently. Go to the bathroom at night only if awakened by the need to go.

2. Days 4–6: Increase the time between emptying your bladder to one and a half hours.

3. Days 7–9: Increase the interval to two hours.

4. Days 10–12: Increase the interval to two and a half hours, and work your way up to emptying your bladder every three to three and a half hours.

It is important, especially in the beginning, to go to the bathroom as close to the proper time as possible. That is, if you are supposed to go at 3:00 p.m., and it is 2:50 p.m. when you feel the urge to go, try to hold it until 3:00 p.m.

BEHAVIORAL STRATEGIES FOR COPING WITH SEXUAL CONCERNS

As previously noted, sexual concerns can stem from physical concerns, cognitive reasons, or behavioral factors. Prior to considering any of these strategies, it is important to see your health care provider to confirm your diagnosis or understanding of what is contributing to your sexual concerns. The strategies you choose may depend on what you find out.

Consistent with the CBT model, certain behavioral strategies can have a positive impact on your physical sensations, your thoughts, and how you feel. The following behavioral strategies can be helpful in addressing sexual concerns.

Apply behavioral strategies for urogenital complaints: If you have concluded that the urogenital problem you are experiencing is contributing to, or resulting in, a sexual concern, you may want to revisit the behavioral strategies listed in this chapter, as well as speak with your health care provider about treatment options. Resolving one problem can have a positive impact on the other.

Target self-image with physical activity and positive lifestyle changes: The physical impact of the menopausal transition and aging in general can have a negative effect on your self-image. However, you may find that positive changes to your lifestyle can make you feel much better about yourself mentally, physically, and sexually. For instance, engaging in more physical activity, regardless of whether weight loss is a motivator for you, as well as tailoring your diet to include more healthy foods, can have a major impact on how you feel about yourself.

Talk to your health care provider: It's important to make sure that you don't have any illnesses that could be contributing to your lack of sexual desire or motivation. If you are already on medication, you may need to ask if it has any potential side effects that might be affecting your libido. This is especially important to do if you have ruled out all other factors for your lack of sex drive.

Apply CBT strategies to cope with hot flashes: The idea of engaging in sexual activity when you know that it could trigger a hot flash or night sweat might lead you to avoid sex altogether. Applying strategies to cope with hot flashes would be helpful in this case. See chapter 5.

Find different times of the day: Oftentimes sexual activity is initiated at night. If fatigue or lack of energy is a factor, or if you are experiencing sleep issues, sexual activity will likely not be a high priority at bedtime. If this is the case, thinking outside the box is necessary along with making sex a priority. For instance, determining when you have more energy in the day, such as first thing in the morning or in the early afternoon, might be helpful in choosing when you will engage in sex. Making sex a priority by planning times to be intimate can also be useful.

Increase communication with your sexual partner: A breakdown in communication can lead to different beliefs and assumptions that are not necessarily true. For example, Ellen stopped all sexual activities with her husband as her belief was that any initiation would lead to painful sexual intercourse. Ellen also felt that her relationship with her husband was in jeopardy because there was no sex. It is important to discuss these things with your partner to clarify whether or not your beliefs are accurate and to potentially negotiate a plan that considers both parties' needs and desires.

Identify what increased your sexual arousal in the past: If you are finding it difficult to become aroused sexually, it might be worthwhile to reflect on what helped in the past. This might mean considering certain environments, planned date nights, certain attire, erotic literature, and so on. If it worked before, chances are it will work again!

Trying something new: This can mean changing anything, from when and where you engage in sexual activity to what you have on when you're intimate. It's all about doing something different that you'd like to try. Novelty can spark arousal. Erotic literature and imagery can also increase the libido.

Choose one or more of these behavioral strategies to try. You can conduct an experiment where you implement one or two strategies at a time and record the results, but be sure to try any new behavior or technique several times before deciding if you found it helpful or not.

Sexual Behavior Modification Experiment

Record when you tried a new behavior or technique, what you tried, and the outcome (Did you notice any change or find the strategy helpful?).

Date	Behavior/Technique Chosen	Outcome

COGNITIVE STRATEGIES FOR COPING WITH SEXUAL CONCERNS

The impact that your thoughts and beliefs can have on your sexual functioning can be striking. Recall some of the thoughts and beliefs that Ellen had recorded in her diary: *Sex will be painful. I am no longer sexually appealing. Our relationship is in jeopardy.* As she was having these thoughts, Ellen withdrew not only from sex but also from any form of intimacy with her husband. Communication between Ellen and her husband began to break down, which resulted in a number of further assumptions that were likely distorted from reality.

This example stresses the importance of examining your own thoughts and beliefs about sex in general, the relationship you have with your partner, and your self-image to determine whether any cognitive distortions are present that you can correct. Keeping a record of your thoughts can help. Note that you do not need to be involved in a sexual or intimate encounter to reflect on your thoughts and beliefs regarding sex. Possibly, your sexual concerns or urogenital problems have led you to avoid being involved in an intimate relationship. If this is the case, you may find that you don't have a specific situation to record, but you can record your thoughts and feelings in general, or you can think about a past situation or an anticipated situation.

The following thought record shows how Ellen did this exercise.

Ellen's Thought Record

Situation	Feelings (0–100)	Thoughts/Predictions	Cognitive Distortions	Alternative Thoughts
Sunday evening cleaning up following dinner. My husband embraces me and I tense up.	anxious (80) guilty (60) depressed (70)	He is going to want to have sex with me, and it will be unbearably painful. I am not fulfilling his needs. I do not have anything to offer anymore. Our relationship is in jeopardy. I am no longer sexually appealing. My sex life is over!	probability overestimation catastrophizing fortune-telling mind reading	My husband doesn't necessarily want to have sex right now. He used to hug me all the time and might just want to show me some affection. Even if we engage in some form of sexual intimacy, it does not have to end in intercourse. He has other needs that I meet that are not sexual. I would probably feel better if I could talk to him about this. My close friend experienced the same problem, and she is now having a better sex life. She encouraged me to see my family doctor for treatment options.

Your Thought Record

Keep a thought record to record and examine your thoughts and predictions about sex. Write down the situation where the thought or prediction occurs. Record your feelings at the time and their intensity on a scale of 0 to 100 (where 0 is the least intense and 100 is the most intense). Record what you were thinking and identify any cognitive distortions (see list in chapter 4). Finally, come up with some alternative, more realistic ways of thinking that will make you feel better.

Situation	Feelings (0–100)	Thoughts/Predictions	Cognitive Distortions	Alternative Thoughts

Bringing It All Together

If you have sexual concerns, whether they began with something physical in nature, such as dysuria or vaginal atrophy, or they are related to poor self-image, there are many strategies you can use to reduce your distress. Once again, you should seek diagnostic clarification with your health care professional to ensure that the treatment plan you have is appropriate. Behavioral and cognitive strategies, introduced in this chapter—used alone or in conjunction with medical or surgical interventions—will help reduce your distress and improve your sexual health.

Overall, it is essential to remain actively aware of how one difficulty or area of distress can lead to others. Something that started out as a urogenital problem, as in Ellen's case, quickly led to sexual concerns with a few very powerful but distorted thoughts and beliefs. Remaining actively aware can allow you to recognize the connections between your thoughts, feelings, behaviors, and physical sensations. You can then make strategic changes that will improve your overall well-being.

SUMMING IT ALL UP

- There are a number of urogenital problems that you may experience during the menopausal transition, including dysuria, urinary incontinence, vaginitis, and vaginal atrophy.

- Common factors that influence urogenital problems during the menopausal transition include a depletion of estrogen, vaginal childbirth, and aging.

- Sexual concerns, such as decreased libido and motivation to engage in sex, are also common during the menopausal transition. Sexual concerns can result from a number of factors: biological, such as hormone fluctuations, psychological, such as personal experiences, and social, including cultural factors.

- It is important to meet with your health care provider so that you can formally diagnose your symptoms and plan appropriate treatment.

- There are a number of treatment options for urogenital problems and sexual concerns, including hormonal, nonhormonal, and behavioral and cognitive strategies.

- You can use both cognitive and behavioral strategies to reduce your distress; these strategies will work either on their own or as a complement to other treatment prescribed by a health care professional.

CHAPTER 10

Consolidating Your Gains and Moving Forward

What do I do next?

How can I continue the work that I have started?

What should I do if I feel like my symptoms are worsening?

How do I move forward in this new phase of my life?

Menopause is a major life transition that can be marked by unpleasant and uncomfortable symptoms. In reading this book, you have gained a deeper understanding of what is happening to your body in response to changing hormone levels and gained greater awareness of how menopausal symptoms have been affecting your life. This knowledge has formed the foundation for strategically managing your symptoms. More specifically, the CBT model has given you a new perspective on your experience, so you can now see your response to situational triggers in terms of the interactions between your thoughts, feelings, physical sensations, and behaviors. This change in how you view your experience is essential to changing your response.

As you worked through this book, you focused on those symptoms that have affected your functioning and quality of life. You learned a range of cognitive and behavioral strategies to target these symptoms, take control, and reduce your discomfort. So what are the next steps? The focus of this final chapter is on helping you maintain your gains and giving you strategies to manage if any of your symptoms should become worse. The final task is to look at the big picture and how to move forward in this new phase of your life.

MAINTAINING YOUR GAINS

We don't expect that your symptoms will have been eliminated completely at this time. The goal of this book is to give you tools to help lessen the intensity of your symptoms and their interference in your life. You may have noticed both a decrease in the intensity of your menopausal symptoms and a decrease in their impact on your day-to-day functioning. This is a success!

For example, in Jane's case, the severity of her hot flashes came down from a rating of 65 to a rating of 30 in intensity and discomfort levels. The interference in her life decreased from a rating of 85 to a rating of 20. She found that she was less anxious and more prepared for the times when she did have a hot flash and that she was in a better position to cope with it. She found such behavioral modifications as dressing in layers and carrying a frozen water bottle in her purse to be helpful. Jane also found the cognitive strategies she'd learned extremely effective for counteracting her negative thoughts related to having hot flashes. She was gradually able to reengage with her life and, as she did so, felt her confidence returning.

The menopausal transition is a process, and you now have the tools that you need to continue to manage your symptoms for as long as you need to. To maintain your gains and to make further gains, you need to keep practicing the CBT strategies you've learned. Assessing your progress at this point will help you identify where you are and where you would like to go. To do this, you may want to consider the intensity and interference of your symptoms during the last week, rate each symptom in terms of its intensity and interference in your life, and then compare this with what you recorded in chapter 2.

Measuring Your Progress

List the menopausal symptom(s) that you recorded on the symptom rating form in chapter 2, along with what you recorded for each symptom's severity and interference. Record these ratings in the "before" column, since they represent how you felt before beginning CBT treatment. Now, using your experience of the last week as a basis, rate each symptom again in terms of how severe or intense it is for you and how much it interferes with your life. Again, rate the symptom's severity (or intensity) on a 0 to 100 scale, where 0 is not at all severe and 100 is the most severe. Then rate the symptom's interference (impact) on a 0 to 100 scale, where 0 is no interference and 100 is the greatest interference.

Symptom Description	Severity/Intensity (0–100) Before	After	Interference/Impact (0–100) Before	After
Example: *hot flashes*	65	30	85	20
1.				
2.				
3.				
4.				
5.				
6.				
7				
8.				

Now take a moment to go back to chapter 4, and reread the goals you made then. Think about how you felt before and after using the treatments in this book. What progress have you made with each of your symptoms? What progress have you made overall? Write down your thoughts in the following space.

Symptom 1: _____

Symptom 2: _____

Symptom 3: _____

Overall progress: _____

What is the most important thing you have learned by working through this book?
_____
_____

What strategies were most helpful?
_____
_____

What do you still need to work on? What are your new goals? Write down your goals for each symptom in the following space:

Symptom 1: _____

Symptom 2: _____

Symptom 3: _____

How will you work on your goals? Write down your plans in the following space:

Symptom 1: _____

Symptom 2: _____

Symptom 3: _____

Consolidating Your Gains and Moving Forward

Now the key is turning your plans into action. You need to make yourself a priority on a daily basis and take time to complete new worksheets or to practice cognitive and behavioral strategies as you need them.

IF YOUR SYMPTOMS GET WORSE

You are in a good position to maintain or even improve on your gains, but what if you suddenly notice a symptom worsening, or you experience a new symptom? This is the time to be proactive and use the techniques you learned in this book to directly target the symptom.

You also may want to consider if stress is a factor, since stress may lead to worsening of symptoms or triggering of new symptoms. Research has shown that stress exacerbates the physical symptoms of menopause and increases the likelihood of mood-related problems during the menopausal transition (Alexander et al. 2007). Although stress is a part of daily life, you can develop skills to manage your stress and reduce the negative effect it can have on your well-being by doing the following:

- Be aware of the causes of stress in your life. The more aware you are, the better positioned you are to take steps to eliminate sources of stress, if possible, or tackle them head on.

- Use the cognitive and behavioral strategies in this book to help you manage stress by addressing cognitive distortions, tackling worries and negative thoughts, and developing action plans to address realistic problems.

- Use mindfulness to cope with stress and improve your general well-being.

The rest of this chapter will help you learn more about mindfulness as a complement to the CBT techniques you've already learned.

PRACTICING MINDFULNESS

Mindfulness, as a new therapeutic approach, has become increasingly popular over the last few decades as a result of accumulating evidence of its effectiveness. Mindfulness-based treatment programs have emerged as a helpful strategy for the reduction of symptoms and distress associated with a number of physical conditions and psychological disorders (Kabat-Zinn 1990; Segal, Williams, and Teasdale 2002).

Mindfulness was traditionally an Asian practice and part of Buddhist culture, but recently Jon Kabat-Zinn, a molecular biologist with a long-term meditation practice, saw the potential for its helpfulness in reducing physical and mental distress. Kabat-Zinn founded the Mindfulness Based Stress Reduction (MBSR) Program at the University of Massachusetts Medical Center, a program proven to be successful with patients suffering from anxiety and chronic pain (Kabat-Zinn et al. 1992). Many health care professionals now refer their patients for training in mindfulness practice to deal better with stress, pain, and illness.

So, what exactly is mindfulness? Mindfulness is a particular attitude toward your experiences, or way of relating to life, that holds the promise of both alleviating your suffering and making your life rich and meaningful (Siegel 2010). It does this by attuning you to your moment-to-moment experience and giving you direct insight into how your mind creates unnecessary anguish. Mindfulness meditation, also known as *insight meditation*, has been formally defined as a nonelaborative, nonjudgmental, present-centered awareness in which each thought, feeling, or sensation that arises in the attentional field is acknowledged and accepted as it is (Kabat-Zinn 1990; Kabat-Zinn, Lipworth, and Burney 1985). In other words, mindfulness is about being fully aware of whatever is happening to you in the present moment. When you are practicing mindfulness, you are cultivating awareness of the mind and body and living in the moment, here and now.

The goal of mindfulness from a therapeutic or clinical perspective can be described as to help you embrace, rather than resist, the inevitable ups and downs of life and equip you to handle the predicaments that everyone experiences from time to time (Siegel 2010). By engaging in mindfulness, you begin to recognize how your habitual thinking patterns, behaviors, and reactivity to sensations, thoughts, and emotions increase your stress and emotional distress. Mindfulness offers a space for you to do this by stepping outside of your mind and simply observing thoughts and other experiences as they come and go.

The ultimate aim is to reduce the vulnerability to these mind states so that, with time, you can learn to acknowledge difficult feelings and thoughts, see their origins more clearly, and experience deeper states of acceptance and peace. Ultimately, you would have a different relationship with the thoughts, feelings, and sensations that make up your everyday experiences, and the result would be an enhancement of your psychological and physical well-being.

As clinicians and patients started to observe the success of MBSR techniques and recognize the link between people's relationships with their thoughts/feelings/sensations and the level of distress they experienced, researchers started to consider other physical and mental health-related problems for which mindfulness could be beneficial. Relapse prevention of depression has emerged as one of these potential applications. A program called mindfulness-based cognitive therapy (MBCT) (Segal, Williams, and Teasdale 2002) was designed for individuals who had suffered from multiple episodes of depression but were currently in remission. This mindfulness treatment approach has been shown to help prevent patients from slipping into further depressive episodes. Mindfulness practices have also been tailored to reduce the symptoms and distress that accompany many other physical problems and mental health disorders, such as chronic pain (Kabat-Zinn, Lipworth, and Burney 1985), stress (Shapiro, Schwartz, and Bonner 1998), panic disorder (Kabat-Zinn et al. 1992), eating disorders (Kristeller and Hallett 1999), suicidal behavior (Linehan et al. 1991), and multiple mental health issues (Green and Bieling 2012).

Menopause and Mindfulness

You may have noticed that throughout this workbook, we emphasized awareness as a way to work toward relief from your menopausal symptoms. Developing awareness meant reflecting on your experiences and thinking about how different variables, such as thoughts, behaviors, and physical sensations, interacted to form those experiences. We stressed that awareness must come first. Only when awareness is present can you make some strategic changes that may help reduce some of the distress you are experiencing. Recall, for instance, chapter 5 on hot flashes. We first promoted awareness by providing information on what is happening to your body, along with tools to help you document your experience with this symptom. We then gave you such tools as thought records and the evidence technique and behavioral modifications to reduce the intensity, distress, and frequency with which you experienced this symptom.

Mindfulness is similar to CBT in that it is a unique practice that facilitates awareness. Although the clinical goal of a mindfulness practice would be the same as CBT, to reduce the distress associated with a symptom, the way mindfulness practice would go about achieving this goal is different. With mindfulness—

instead of trying to change your thoughts and behaviors—you would cultivate a different relationship with your experiences in terms of the thoughts, feelings, or sensations that you have.

Recently, a group of researchers (Carmody et al. 2011) advocated the benefits of mindfulness training for coping with hot flashes. They implemented an eight-week mindfulness-based training program, consistent with Kabat-Zinn's MBSR techniques, to determine if women could feel less bothered by their hot flashes. As you can see, the goal was not necessarily to reduce the experience of hot flashes in terms of frequency or intensity. Instead, the mindfulness practice aimed to change how these women experienced their hot flashes, namely to reduce the distress associated with their symptoms. The results indicated that mindfulness could be an effective therapeutic strategy to reduce distress associated with hot flashes and night sweats; its beneficial effects were maintained long after the mindfulness program ended and led to other improvements, related to anxiety, quality of sleep, and quality of life. Given these results, you may want to consider exploring mindfulness as yet another complementary therapeutic approach for relief of your menopausal symptoms.

The following mindfulness exercise comes from *A Mindfulness-Based Stress Reduction Workbook* (Stahl and Goldstein 2010, 18–19). This exercise involves mindfully eating a raisin, though any food will suffice if eaten in this manner. Before beginning, you should put aside anything else that you've been doing and eliminate all distractions, such as the phone, TV, or radio. The goal is to focus your full attention on the experience.

Mindfully Eating a Raisin

Place a few raisins in your hand. If you don't have raisins, any food will do. Imagine that you have just come to Earth from a distant planet without such food.

Now, with this food in hand, you can begin to explore it with all of your senses.

Focus on one of the objects as if you've never seen anything like it before. Focus on seeing this object. Scan it, exploring every part of it, as if you've never seen such a thing before. Turn it around with your fingers and notice what color it is.

Notice the folds and where the surface reflects light or becomes darker.

Next, explore the texture, feeling any softness, hardness, coarseness, or smoothness.

While you're doing this, if thoughts arise such as "Why am I doing this weird exercise?" "How will this ever help me?" or "I hate these objects," then just see if you can acknowledge these thoughts, let them be, and then bring your awareness back to the object.

Take the object beneath your nose and carefully notice the smell of it.

Bring the object to one ear, squeeze it, roll it around, and hear if there is any sound coming from it.

Begin to slowly take the object to your mouth, noticing how the arm knows exactly where to go and perhaps becoming aware of your mouth watering.

Gently place the object in your mouth, on your tongue, without biting it. Simply explore the sensations of this object in your mouth.

When you're ready, intentionally bite down on the object, maybe noticing how it automatically goes to one side of the mouth versus the other. Also notice the tastes it releases.

Slowly chew this object. Be aware of the saliva in your mouth and how the object changes in consistency as you chew.

When you feel ready to swallow, consciously notice the intention to swallow, then see if you can notice the sensations of swallowing the raisin, sensing it moving down to your throat and into your esophagus on its way to your stomach.

Take a moment to congratulate yourself for taking this time to experience mindful eating.

Reflecting on Your Mindful Experience

After doing this mindfulness meditation, take a couple minutes to reflect on your experience. Was there anything different or surprising about this experience compared to how you have eaten raisins in the past? Reflect on all aspects of your sensory experience. What did you notice about your thoughts? Write down your observations in the following space:

_____
_____
_____
_____
_____
_____
_____

If you would like to develop a mindfulness practice or learn more about mindfulness, the suggested reading section at the end of this book includes some excellent resources.

MOVING ON, MOVING FORWARD

Menopause is a major life transition that may evoke much self-reflection. You may wonder about what this means for you, your identity, your life, and your future. You will recall that for Catherine, menopause was associated with introspection and questioning the meaning of her life. She questioned whether she had made the right decision in not having children, as the onset of menopause made this decision final. Not surprisingly, her main symptom related to menopause was depression. Catherine worked hard at implementing the strategies from chapter 7. She found that cognitive and behavioral strategies helped her work through her negative thoughts and focus on what was important to her, especially her family relationships and her work as a teacher. She was able to reframe how she viewed herself and her future in a more helpful and adaptive way. As a result, Catherine was able to move forward with greater confidence in her decisions and with a positive view on the future.

In preparing to write this book, we surveyed many women in various stages of the menopausal transition. Like Catherine, some women reported that menopause led them to some deep reflections on themselves and the future. As one respondent said, "Arriving at menopause did bring with it a bit of a sense of loss. Fertility is so associated with femininity that I have to admit, once menopause occurred, I wondered if I was somehow less feminine. It's also the end of a stage of life, perhaps the beginning of the final stage of life. That's quite a heavy thought and certainly gives food for contemplation."

In dealing with the negative effects of menopause, survey respondents also spoke about their strategies for coping. Their responses reflected some common themes as they spoke of making positive adjustments.

Newfound Freedom

Some women discovered a new sense of freedom at this stage of life with the end of menses: "I was glad to put my menses behind me." "It was nice not having to deal with my monthly visitor." "I could engage in any activity, like swimming, and not have to worry about it." "It was nice to be free of the need for feminine hygiene products."

Increased Confidence and Wisdom

Some women focused on the positives of the aging process, such as the increased confidence and wisdom they noticed in themselves. One woman said, "When I got to menopause, I was heavily into women's spirituality, and so I considered that menopause is the beginning of the Crone Age, where woman keeps her wise blood and becomes even more free to do as she will. I love my body, even as I noticed that I have to work a little harder at keeping fit, but that's okay." Another woman wrote, "Although I worry about the stigma attached to aging, the wisdom and confidence I have are better than I have ever been. There is clarity that comes with this age. I am looking forward to full menopause—just have to get through the body not knowing what it wants to do."

Valuing Positive Relationships

The importance of friendships was a common theme: "I have been blessed with lifelong relationships. I cherish my friends, and invest time, energy, and spirit into nurturing these. As time goes on, my relationships are all the more precious." "I used my friends for support as they were going through the same thing—we would laugh about the embarrassing moments."

Keeping Up Your Interests

Women spoke of not letting menopause stop them from doing the activities that were important to them or that they wanted to do. One woman commented, "I just kept plugging along." Another said, "I do what I love to do and keep busy doing what I love to do: traveling, visiting friends and family, writing."

Maintaining a Balanced and Positive Attitude

Finally, many women expressed a balanced and optimistic outlook: "In the end, menopause is just that…a transition. It is a change, but there are certainly much, much worse things in life. All changes need to be approached with a positive attitude and a sense of humor. That's what I've tried to do!"

WELL-BEING DURING MIDLIFE AND BEYOND

Working through this book, you have taken a direct and adaptive approach to coping with some negative effects of menopause. The good news is that the CBT skills you've developed can be applied to the larger process of aging.

This book has spent a significant amount of time reviewing strategies for tackling symptoms, thoughts, and behaviors associated with your current stage in life. We wanted to end by dedicating a few lines to looking ahead and providing some ideas on a healthier way to approach the late postmenopausal years, in your sixties, seventies, eighties, and—why not?—nineties.

An issue often discussed by patients and health professionals is the desire to remain cognitively healthy later in life: the desire to remain sharp and avoid the deterioration of memory and attention or to avoid dementia. As you grow older, you may notice that your cognitive abilities are not as they once were. This experience was captured by one of our survey respondents: "It seems my memory may not be as sharp at times. It takes longer sometimes to come up with a word or a name. That is frustrating. I'm not even certain it is a result of menopause. It may be aging in general, being extremely busy, or some other reason. But menopause is a convenient excuse!"

Although the clinical characteristics and possible causes of dementia and cognitive decline are multiple and complex, some recent studies have shown how science sometimes simply reinforces common sense. These studies associate healthy lifestyle practices, such as regular exercise, intellectual activity, social relationships, and a healthy diet, with a modest reduction in risk for dementia, including Alzheimer's disease, even among those participants at higher risk due to family history (Baker et al. 2012; Deweerdt 2011). Thus, you have now a few more reasons to eat healthier, to remain socially engaged, and to stay physically and mentally active throughout the years.

Suggested Reading

Feeling Good: The New Mood Therapy. By David D. Burns. New York: William Morrow, 1980.

Full Catastrophe Living: Using the Wisdom of Your Body and Mind to Face Stress, Pain, and Illness. By Jon Kabat-Zinn. New York: Delacorte, 1990.

The Menopausal Transition: Interface between Psychiatry and Gynecology (Key Issues in Mental Health). Edited by Claudio N. Soares and Michelle P. Warren. Basel, Switzerland: S. Karger Publishers, 2009.

Mind over Mood: Changing How You Feel by Changing the Way You Think. By Dennis Greenberger and Christine A. Padesky. London: Guilford Press, 1995.

The Mindful Way through Depression: Freeing Yourself from Chronic Unhappiness. By Mark Williams, John Teasdale, Zindel Segal, and Jon Kabat-Zinn. New York: Guilford Press, 2007.

A Mindfulness-Based Stress Reduction Workbook. By Bob Stahl and Elisha Goldstein. Oakland: New Harbinger Publications, 2010.

The Mindfulness Solution: Everyday Practices for Everyday Problems. By Ronald D. Siegel. New York: Guilford Press, 2010.

Phobic Disorders and Panic in Adults: A Guide to Assessment and Treatment. By Martin M. Antony and Richard P. Swinson. Washington, DC: American Psychological Association, 2000.

References

Abdali, K., M. Khajehei, and H. R. Tabatabaee. 2010. "Effect of St. John's Wort on Severity, Frequency, and Duration of Hot Flashes in Premenopausal, Perimenopausal and Postmenopausal Women: A Randomized, Double-Blind, Placebo-Controlled Study." *Menopause* 17: 326.

Albertazzi, P. 2007. "Non-Estrogenic Approaches for the Treatment of Climacteric Symptoms." *Climacteric* 10 (Suppl. 2): 115–20.

Alexander, J. L., L. Dennerstein, N. F. Woods, B. S. McEwen, U. Halbreich, K. Kotz, and G. Richardson. 2007. "Role of Stressful Life Events and Menopausal Stage in Well-Being and Health." *Expert Review of Neurotherapeutics* 7: S93–S113.

American Psychiatric Association 2000. *Diagnostic and Statistical Manual of Mental Disorders (DSM-IV-TR)*. 4th ed., text rev. Washington, DC: American Psychiatric Association.

Antony, M. M., and R. P. Swinson. 2000. *Phobic Disorders and Panic in Adults: A Guide to Assessment and Treatment*. Washington, DC: American Psychological Association.

Archer, D. F., L. Seidman, G. D. Constantine, J. H. Pickar, and S. Olivier. 2009. "A Double-Blind, Randomly Assigned, Placebo-Controlled Study of Desvenlafaxine Efficacy and Safety for the Treatment of Vasomotor Symptoms Associated with Menopause." *American Journal of Obstetrics and Gynecology* 200: 172.e1–172.e10.

Baker, L. D., J. L. Bayer-Carter, J. Skinner, T. J. Montine, B. A. Cholerton, M. Callaghan, J. Leverenz, B. K. Walter, E. Tsai, N. Postupna, J. Lampe, and S. Craft. 2012. "High-Intensity Physical Activity Modulates Diet Effects on Cerebrospinal Amyloid-ß Levels in Normal Aging and Mild Cognitive Impairment." *Journal of Alzheimer's Disease* 28 (1): 137–46.

Barlow, D. H., and M. G. Craske. 1994. *Mastery of Your Anxiety and Panic II*. Albany, NY: Graywind Publications.

Beck, A. T., A. J. Rush, B. F. Shaw, and G. Emery. 1979. *Cognitive Therapy of Depression*. New York: Guilford Press.

Bo, K., R. H. Hagen, B. Kvarstein, J. Jorgensen, and S. Laresen. 1990. "Pelvic Floor Muscle Exercise for the Treatment of Female Stress Urinary Incontinence: III. Effects of Two Different Degrees of Pelvic Floor Muscle Exercises." *Neurourology Urodynamics* 9: 489–502.

Bonnet, M. B. 2005. "Burden of Chronic Insomnia on the Individual." Paper presented at NIH State-of-the-Science Conference on Manifestations and Management of Chronic Insomnia in Adults, Bethesda, MD, June 13.

Borud, E. K., T. Alraek, A. White, and S. Grimsgaard. 2010. "The Acupuncture on Hot Flashes among Menopausal Women Study: Observational Follow-Up Results at Six and Twelve Months." *Menopause* 17: 262–68.

Bromberger, J. T., and H. M. Kravitz. 2011. "Mood and Menopause: Findings from the Study of Women's Health across the Nation (SWAN) over Ten Years." *Obstetrics and Gynecology Clinics of North America* 38: 609–25.

Burns, D. D. 1980. *Feeling Good: The New Mood Therapy*. New York: William Morrow.

Buster, J. E. 2010. "Transdermal Menopausal Hormone Therapy: Delivery through Skin Changes the Rules." *Expert Opinion on Pharmacotherapy* 11 (9): 1489–1499.

Butler, A. C., J. E. Chapman, E. M. Forman, and A. T. Beck. 2006. "The Empirical Status of Cognitive-Behavioral Therapy: A Review of Meta-Analyses." *Clinical Psychology Review* 26: 17–31.

Cardoso, C. G. Jr., F. C. Rosas, B. Oneda, E. Labes, T. Tinucci, S. B. Abrahão SB, A. M. da Fonseca, D. Mion Jr., and C. L. Forjaz. 2011. "Aerobic Training Abolishes Ambulatory Blood Pressure Increase Induced by Estrogen Therapy: A Double Blind Randomized Clinical Trial." *Maturitas* 69 (2): 189–194.

Carmody, J. F., S. Crawford, E. Salmoirago-Blotcher, K. Leung, L. Churchill, and N. Olendzki. 2011. "Mindfulness Training for Coping with Hot Flashes: Results of a Randomized Trial." *Menopause* 18: 611–20.

Carney, C. E., and R. Manber. 2009. *How to Quiet Your Mind and Get to Sleep: Solutions to Insomnia for Those with Depression, Anxiety, or Chronic Pain*. Oakland, CA: New Harbinger Publications.

Carney, C. E., and W. F. Waters. 2006. "Effects of a Structured Problem-Solving Procedure on Pre-Sleep Cognitive Arousal in College Students with Insomnia." *Behavioral Sleep Medicine* 4: 13–28.

Cohen, L. S., C. N. Soares, A. F. Vitonis, M. W. Otto, and B. L. Harlow. 2006. "Risk for New Onset of Depression during the Menopausal Transition: The Harvard Study of Moods and Cycles." *Archives of General Psychiatry* 63: 385–90.

Col, N. F., J. R. Guthrie, M. Politi, and L. Dennerstein. 2009. "Duration of Vasomotor Symptoms in Middle-Aged Women: A Longitudinal Study." *Menopause* 16: 453–57.

Colgan, R., and M. Williams. 2011. "Diagnosis and Treatment of Acute Uncomplicated Cystitis." *American Family Physician* 84: 771–76.

Deweerdt, S. 2011. "Prevention: Activity Is the Best Medicine." *Nature* 475: S16–17.

Dorsey, C. M., K. A. Lee, and M. B. Scharf. 2004. "Effect of Zolpidem on Sleep in Women with Perimenopausal and Postmenopausal Insomnia: A Four-Week, Randomized, Multicenter, Double-Blind, Placebo-Controlled Study." *Clinical Therapy* 26: 1578–88.

Eichling, P. S. 2002. "Evaluating and Treating Menopausal Sleep Problems." *Menopause Management* 11: 8–17.

Ellis, A., and R. A. Harper. 1961. *A Guide to Rational Living*. Englewood Cliffs, NJ: Prentice-Hall.

Evans, M. L., E. Pritts, E. Vittinghoff, K. McClish, K. S. Morgan, and R. B. Jaffe. 2005. "Management of Postmenopausal Hot Flashes with Venlafaxine Hydrochloride: A Randomized Controlled Trial." *Obstetrics and Gynecology* 105: 161–66.

Freedman, R. R. 2005. "Hot Flashes: Behavioral Treatments, Mechanisms, and Relation to Sleep." *American Journal of Medicine* 118: 124–30.

Freedman, R. R., D. Norton, S. Woodward, and G. Cornelissen. 1995. "Core Body Temperature and Circadian Rhythm of Hot Flashes in Menopausal Women." *Journal of Clinical Endocrinology and Metabolism* 80: 2354–2358.

Freedman, R. R., and T. A. Roehrs. 2004. "Lack of Sleep Disturbance from Menopausal Hot Flashes." *Fertility and Sterility* 82: 138–144.

———. 2007. "Sleep Disturbance in Menopause." *Menopause* 14: 826–29.

Freedman, R. R., and S. Woodward. 1992. "Behavioral Treatment of Menopausal Hot Flushes: Evaluation by Ambulatory Monitoring." *American Journal of Obstetrics and Gynecology* 167: 436–39.

Freeman, E. W., K. A. Guthrie, B. Caan, B. Sternfeld, L. S. Cohen, H. Joffe, J. S. Carpenter, G. L. Anderson, J. C. Larson, K. E. Ensrud, S. D. Reed, K. M. Newton, S. Sherman, M. D. Samuel, and A. Z. LaCroix. 2011. "Efficacy of Escitalopram for Hot Flashes in Healthy Menopausal Women." *Journal of the American Medical Association* 305: 267–74.

Freeman, E. W., and K. Sherif. 2007. "Prevalence of Hot Flushes and Night Sweats around the World: A Systematic Review." *Climacteric* 10: 197–214.

Freeman, M. P., J. R. Hibbeln, M. Silver, A. M. Hirschberg, B. Wang, A. M. Yule, L. F. Petrillo, E. Pascuillo, N. I. Economou, H. Joffe, and L. S. Cohen. 2011. "Omega-3 Fatty Acids for Major Depressive Disorder Associated with the Menopausal Transition: A Preliminary Open Trial." *Menopause* 18: 279–84.

Frey, B. N., C. Lord, and C. N. Soares. 2008. "Depression during Menopausal Transition: A Review of Treatment Strategies and Pathophysiological Correlates." *Menopause International* 14: 123–28.

Gold, E. B., B. Sternfeld, and J. L. Kelsey. 2000. "Relation of Demographic and Lifestyle Factors to Symptoms in a Multi-Racial/Ethnic Population of Women Forty to Fifty-Five Years of Age." *American Journal of Epidemiology* 152: 463–73.

Gomelsky, A., and R. R. Dmochowski. 2011. "Treatment of Mixed Urinary Incontinence in Women." *Current Opinion in Obstetrics and Gynecology* 23: 371–75.

Gordon, P. R., J. P. Kerwin, K. J. Boesen, and J. Senf. 2006. "Sertraline to Treat Hot Flashes: A Randomized Controlled Double Blind, Crossover Trial in a General Population." *Menopause* 13: 568–75.

Green, S. M., and P. J. Bieling. 2012. "Expanding the Scope of Mindfulness-Based Cognitive Therapy: Evidence for Effectiveness in a Heterogeneous Psychiatric Sample." *Cognitive and Behavioral Practice* 19: 174–80.

Green, S. M., E. Haber, R. E. McCabe, and C. N. Soares. 2010. "Cognitive-Behavioural Group Treatment (CBGT) for Menopausal Symptoms: A Pilot Study." Paper presented at the Association for Behavioral and Cognitive Therapies, San Francisco, November.

Guimarães, A. C. A., and F. Baptista. 2011. "Influence of Habitual Physical Activity on the Symptoms of Climacterium/Menopause and the Quality of Life of Middle-Aged Women." *International Journal of Women's Health* 3: 319–28.

Hall, E., B. N. Frey, and C. N. Soares. 2011. "Non-Hormonal Treatment Strategies for Vasomotor Symptoms: A Critical Review." *Drugs* 71: 287–304.

Harman, S. M., E. Vittinghoff, E. A. Brinton, M. J. Budoff, M. I. Cedars, R. A. Lobo, G. R. Merriam, V. M. Miller, F. Naftolin, L. Pal, N. Santoro, H. S. Taylor, and H. M. Black. 2011. "Timing and Duration of Menopausal Hormone Treatment May Affect Cardiovascular Outcomes." *American Journal of Medicine* 124: 199–205.

Harvey, A. G. 2000. "Sleep Hygiene and Sleep-Onset Insomnia." *Journal of Nervous Mental Disorders* 188: 53–55.

Harvey, A. G., and C. Farrell. 2003. "The Efficacy of a Pennebaker-Like Writing Intervention for Poor Sleepers." *Behavioral Sleep Medicine* 1: 115–23.

Hillard, T. 2010. "The Menopausal Bladder." *Menopause International* 16 (2): 74–80.

Hunskaar, S., E. P. Arnold, K. Burgio, A. C. Diokno, A. R. Herzog, and V. T. Mallett. 2000. "Epidemiology and Natural History of Urinary Incontinence." *International Urogynecology Journal* 11: 301–19.

Jacobs, G. D., E. F. Pace-Schott, R. Stickgold, and M. W. Otto. 2004. "Cognitive Behavior Therapy and Pharmacotherapy for Insomnia: A Randomized Controlled Trial and Direct Comparison." *Archives of Internal Medicine* 164: 1888.

Jacobson, N. S., K. S. Dobson, P. A. Truax, M. E. Addis, K. Koerner, J. K. Gollan, E. Gortner, and S. E. Prince. 1996. "A Component Analysis of Cognitive-Behavioral Treatment for Depression." *Journal of Consulting and Clinical Psychology* 64 (2): 295–304.

Joffe, H., C. N. Soares, and L. S. Cohen. 2003. "Assessment and Treatment of Hot Flushes and Menopausal Mood Disturbance." *Psychiatric Clinics of North America* 26 (3): 563–80.

References

Kabat-Zinn, J. 1990. *Full Catastrophe Living: Using the Wisdom of Your Body and Mind to Face Stress, Pain, and Illness*. New York: Delacorte.

Kabat-Zinn, J., L. Lipworth, and R. Burney. 1985. "The Clinical Use of Mindfulness Meditation for the Self-Regulation of Chronic Pain." *Journal of Behavioral Medicine* 8: 163–90.

Kabat-Zinn, J., A. O. Massion, J. Kristeller, L. G. Peterson, K. E. Fletcher, L. Pbert, W. R. Lenderking, and S. F. Santorelli. 1992. "Effectiveness of a Meditation-Based Stress Reduction Program in the Treatment of Anxiety Disorders." *American Journal of Psychiatry* 149: 936–43.

Kessler, R. C., P. Berglund, O. Demler, R. Jin, K. R. Merikangas, and E. E. Walters. 2005. "Lifetime Prevalence and Age-of-Onset Distributions of DSM-IV Disorders in the National Comorbidity Survey Replication." *Archives of General Psychiatry* 62: 593–602.

Kim, K. H., K. W. Kang, D. I. Kim, H. J. Kim, H. M. Yoon, J. M. Lee, J. C. Jeong, M. S. Lee, H. J. Jung, and S. M. Choi. 2010. "Effects of Acupuncture on Hot Flashes in Perimenopausal and Postmenopausal Women: A Multicentre Randomized Clinical Trial." *Menopause* 17: 269–80.

Knight, D. C., J. B. Howes, and J. A. Eden. 1999. "The Effect of Promensil, an Isoflavone Extract, on Menopausal Symptoms." *Climacteric* 2: 79–84.

Kristeller, J. L., and B. Hallett. 1999. "Effects of a Meditation-Based Intervention in the Treatment of Binge Eating." *Journal of Health Psychology* 4: 357–63.

Kronenberg, F. 1990. "Hot Flashes: Epidemiology and Physiology." *Annals of the New York Academy of Sciences* 592: 52–86.

Kronenberg, F., and R. M. Barnard. 1992. "Modulation of Menopausal Hot Flashes by Ambient Temperature." *Journal of Thermal Biology* 17: 43–49.

Krystal, A. D. 2004. "Depression and Insomnia in Women." *Clinical Cornerstone* 6 (S1B): S19–S28.

Landolt, H. P., E. Werth, A. A. Borbély, and D. J. Dijk. 1995. "Caffeine Intake (200 mg) in the Morning Affects Human Sleep and EEG Power Spectra at Night." *Brain Research* 675: 67–74.

Lindau, S. T., L. P. Schumm, E. O. Laumann, W. Levinson, C. A. O'Muircheartaigh, and L. J. Waite. 2007. "A Study of Sexuality and Health among Older Adults in the United States." *New England Journal of Medicine* 357: 762–74.

Linehan, M. M., H. E. Armstrong, A. Saurez, D. Allmon, and H. L. Heard. 1991. "Cognitive-Behavioural Treatment of Chronically Parasuicidal Borderline Patients." *Archives of General Psychiatry* 48: 1060–64.

Lokuge, S., B. N. Frey, J. A. Foster, C. N. Soares, and M. Steiner. 2011. "Depression in Women: Windows of Vulnerability and New Insights into the Link between Estrogen and Serotonin." *Journal of Clinical Psychiatry* 72: e1563–69.

Lukacz, E. S., C. Sampselle, M. Gray, S. Macdiarmid, M. Rosenberg, P. Ellsworth, and M. H. Palmer. 2011. "A Healthy Bladder: A Consensus Statement." *International Journal of Clinical Practice* 65: 1026–36.

Mehta, A., and G. Bachmann. 2008. "Vulvovaginal Complaints." *Clinical Obstetrics and Gynecology* 51: 549–55.

Nappi, R. E., F. Albani, V. Santamaria, S. Tonani, F. Magri, E. Martini, L. Chiovato, and F. Polatti. 2010. "Hormonal and Psycho-Relational Aspects of Sexual Function during Menopausal Transition and at Early Menopause." *Maturitas* 67: 78–83.

National Institutes of Health. 2005. "State-of-the-Science Conference Statement: Management of Menopause-Related Symptoms." *Annals of Internal Medicine* 142 (12): 1003–13.

National Sleep Foundation. 2010. "2007 Women and Sleep." National Sleep Foundation. Accessed October 12. http://www.sleepfoundation.org/article/sleep-america-polls/2007-women-and-sleep.

Newton, K. M., S. D. Reed, A. Z. LaCroix, L. C. Grothaus, and K. Ehrlich. 2006. "Treatment of Vasomotor Symptoms of Menopause with Black Cohosh, Multibotanicals, Soy, Hormone Therapy, or Placebo: A Randomized Trial." *Annals of Internal Medicine* 145: 869–79.

North American Menopause Society. 2007. "The Role of Local Vaginal Estrogen for Treatment of Vaginal Atrophy in Postmenopausal Women: 2007 Position Statement of the North American Menopause Society." *Menopause* 14: 357–69.

———. 2010a. "Estrogen and Progestogen Use in Postmenopausal Women: 2010 Position Statement of the North American Menopause Society." *Menopause* 17: 242–55.

———. 2010b. *Menopause Practice: A Clinician's Guide*. 4th ed. Mayfield Heights, OH: North American Menopause Society.

Palacios, S. 2009. "Managing Urogenital Atrophy." *Maturitas* 63: 315–18.

Randolph, J. F., M. Sowers, E. B. Gold, B. A. Mohr, J. Luborsky, N. Santoro, D. S. McConnell, J. S. Finkelstein, S. G. Korenman, K. A. Matthews, B. Sternfeld, and B. L. Lasley. 2003. "Reproductive Hormones in the Early Menopausal Transition: Relationship to Ethnicity, Body Size, and Menopausal Status." *Journal of Clinical Endocrinology and Metabolism* 88: 1516–22.

Robinson, D., and L. Cardozo. 2011. "Estrogens and the Lower Urinary Tract." *Neurourology and Urodynamics* 30: 754–57.

Rossouw, J. E., G. L. Anderson, R. L. Prentice, A. Z. LaCroix, C. Kooperberg, M. L. Stefanick, R. D. Jackson, S. A. Beresford, B. V. Howard, K. C. Johnson, J. M. Kotchen, and J. Ockene; Writing Group for the Women's Health Initiative Investigators. 2002. "Risks and Benefits of Estrogen Plus Progestin in Healthy Postmenopausal Women: Principal Results from the Women's Health Initiative Randomized Controlled Trial." *Journal of the American Medical Association* 288: 321–33.

Segal, Z. V., J. M. G. Williams, and J. D. Teasdale. 2002. *Mindfulness Based Cognitive Therapy for Depression: A New Approach to Preventing Relapse*. New York: Guilford Press.

Shapiro, S. L., G. E. Schwartz, and G. Bonner. 1998. "Effects of Mindfulness-Based Stress Reduction on Medical or Premedical Students." *Journal of Behavioral Medicine* 21: 581–99.

Siegel, R. D. 2010. *The Mindfulness Solution: Everyday Practices for Everyday Problems*. New York: Guilford Press.

Soares, C. N. 2010. "Can Depression Be a Menopause-Associated Risk?" *BMC Medicine* 8: 79.

Soares, C. N., and B. F. Frey. 2010. "Psychopharmacology for the Clinician." *Journal of Psychiatry and Neuroscience* 35: E6–E7.

Soares, C. N., H. Joffe, R. Rubens, J. Caron, T. Roth, and L. Cohen. 2006. "Eszopiclone in Patients with Insomnia during Perimenopause and Early Postmenopause: A Randomized Controlled Trial." *Obstetrics and Gynecology* 108: 1402–10.

Soares, C. N., and B. J. Murray. 2006. "Sleep Disorders in Women: Clinical Evidence and Treatment Strategies." *Psychiatry Clinics of North America* 29: 1095–1113.

Soares, C. N., and B. Zitek. 2008. "Reproductive Hormone Sensitivity and Risk for Depression across the Female Life Cycle: A Continuum of Vulnerability?" *Journal of Psychiatry and Neuroscience* 33: 331–43.

Soules, M. R., S. Sherman, E. Parrott, R. Rebar, N. Santoro, W. Utian, and N. Woods. 2001. "Executive Summary: Stages of Reproductive Aging Workshop (STRAW) Park City, Utah, July 2001." *Menopause* 8: 402–7.

Stahl, B., and E. Goldstein. 2010. *A Mindfulness-Based Stress Reduction Workbook*. Oakland, CA: New Harbinger Publications.

Stearns, V., K. L. Beebe, M. Iyengar, and E. Dube. 2003. "Paroxetine Controlled Release in the Treatment of Menopausal Hot Flashes: A Randomized Controlled Trial." *Journal of the American Medical Association* 289: 2827–34.

Sturdee, D. W., and N. Panay. 2010. "Recommendations for the Management of Postmenopausal Vaginal Atrophy." *Climacteric* 13: 509–22.

Suvanto-Luukkonen, E., R. Koivunen, H. Sundstrom, R. Bloigu, E. Karjalainen, L. Haiva-Mallinen, and J. S. Tapanainen. 2005. "Citalopram and Fluoxetine in the Treatment of Postmenopausal Symptoms: A Prospective, Randomized Nine-Month, Placebo-Controlled, Double-Blind Study." *Menopause* 12: 18–26.

Teede, H. J. 2007. "Sex Hormones and the Cardiovascular System: Effects on Arterial Function in Women." *Clinical and Experimental Pharmacology and Physiology* 34: 672–76.

Tice, J. A., B. Ettinger, K. Ensrud, W. Wallace, T. Blackwell, and S. R. Cummings. 2003. "Phytoestrogen Supplements for the Treatment of Hot Flashes: The Isoflavone Clover Extract (ICE) Study. A Randomized Controlled Trial." *Journal of the American Medical Association* 290: 207–14.

Warren, M. P. 2004. "A Comparative Review of the Risks and Benefits of Hormone Replacement Therapy Regimens." *American Journal of Obstetrics and Gynecology* 190: 1141–67.

Waters, W. F., M. J. Hurry, P. G. Binks, C. E. Carney, L. E. Lajos, K. H. Fuller, B. Betz, J. Johnson, T. Anderson, and J. M. Tucci. 2003. "Behavioral and Hypnotic Treatments for Insomnia Sub-Types." *Behavioral Sleep Medicine* 1: 81–101.

WHO Scientific Group. 1996. "Research on the Menopause in the 1990s. Report of a WHO Scientific Group." *WHO Technical Report Series* 866: 1–107.

World Health Organization. 2012. "Health Topics: Sexual Health." World Health Organization. Accessed April 18. http://www.who.int/topics/sexual_health/en/.

Woodward, S., and R. R. Freeman. 1994. "The Thermoregulatory Effects of Menopausal Hot Flashes on Sleep." *Sleep* 17: 497–501.

Young, T., M. Palta, J. Dempsey, J. Skatrud, S. Weber, and S. Badr. 1993. "The Occurrence of Sleep-Disordered Breathing among Middle-Aged Adults." New England Journal of Medicine 28: 1230–35.

Sheryl M. Green, PhD, is a clinical health psychologist within the Women's Health Concerns Clinic and Consultation Liaison service at St. Joseph's Healthcare Hamilton in Ontario, Canada. She is also assistant professor in the department of psychiatry and Behavioural Neurosciences at McMaster University in Ontario, Canada.

Randi E. McCabe, PhD, is psychologist-in-chief and director of the Anxiety Treatment and Research Centre at St. Joseph's Healthcare Hamilton. She is also associate professor in the department of psychiatry and behavioural neurosciences at McMaster University in Ontario, Canada.

Claudio N. Soares, MD, PhD, is a psychiatrist and director of the Women's Health Concerns Clinic at St. Joseph's Healthcare Hamilton. He is also the academic head of the mood and anxiety disorders division and professor within the departments of psychiatry and behavioural neurosciences and obstetrics and gynecology at McMaster University in Ontario, Canada.

MORE BOOKS *from* NEW HARBINGER PUBLICATIONS

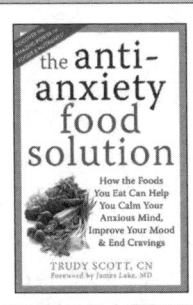

THE ANTI-ANXIETY FOOD SOLUTION
How the Foods You Eat Can Help You Calm Your Anxious Mind, Improve Your Mood & End Cravings
US $17.95 / ISBN: 978-1572249257
Also available as an e-book at newharbinger.com

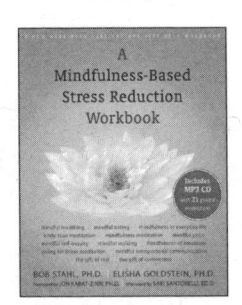

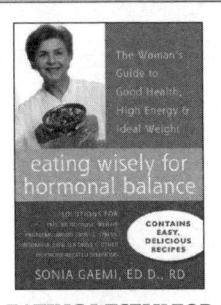

EATING WISELY FOR HORMONAL BALANCE
The Woman's Guide to Good Health, High Energy & Ideal Weight
US $21.95 / ISBN: 978-1572243736
Also available as an e-book at newharbinger.com

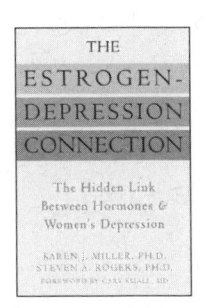

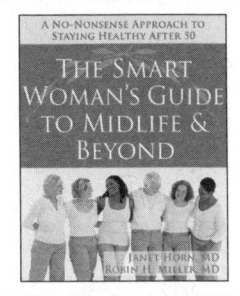

THE SMART WOMAN'S GUIDE TO MIDLIFE & BEYOND
A No-Nonsense Approach to Staying Healthy After 50
US $19.95 / ISBN: 978-1572245563
Also available as an e-book at newharbinger.com

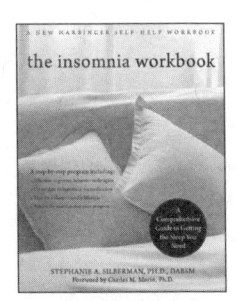

A MINDFULNESS-BASED STRESS REDUCTION WORKBOOK
US $24.95 / ISBN: 978-1572247086
Also available as an e-book at newharbinger.com

THE ESTROGEN-DEPRESSION CONNECTION
The Hidden Link Between Hormones & Women's Depression
US $16.95 / ISBN: 978-157224-4832
Also available as an e-book at newharbinger.com

THE INSOMNIA WORKBOOK
A Comprehensive Guide to Getting the Sleep You Need
US $21.95 / ISBN: 978-1572246355
Also available as an e-book at newharbinger.com

newharbingerpublications, inc.
1-800-748-6273 / newharbinger.com

Like us on Facebook
Follow us on Twitter @newharbinger

(VISA, MC, AMEX / prices subject to change without notice)

Don't miss out on new books in the subjects that interest you.
Sign up for our **Book Alerts** at nhpubs.com/bookalerts

ARE YOU SEEKING A CBT THERAPIST?

The Association for Behavioral & Cognitive Therapies (ABCT) Find-a-Therapist service offers a list of therapists schooled in CBT techniques. Therapists listed are licensed professionals who have met the membership requirements of ABCT & who have chosen to appear in the directory.

Please visit www.abct.org & click on *Find a Therapist*.